letters to the — EXPECTING mama

Published by Goose Water Press LLC.
www.kristenemilybehl.com

For bulk ordering, please email
connect@kristenemilybehl.com.

Copyediting by Daniel Madson (Skrive Publications).
www.skrivepublications.com

Cover design and formatting by David Miles.
www.daviddesignsbooks.com

Doodle art by Anne Loppnow.

ISBN:
E-book 978-1-954809-00-0
Paperback 978-1-954809-01-7
Hardcover 978-1-954809-02-4
Audiobook 978-1-954809-03-1

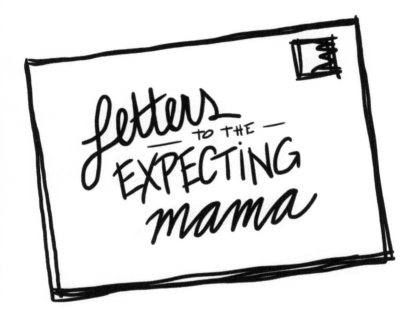

KRISTEN EMILY BEHL

Contents

A Note from Me to You

NOTHING CAN TOUCH YOUR HEART LIKE A handwritten letter. You know that feeling. Someone has taken the time to grab a piece of paper and write a message just for you. Someone has tracked down your address, paid for a stamp, walked to the mailbox or driven to the post office, and mailed it. Someone has waited patiently until the letter arrives days later.

When it finally shows up in your mailbox, how happy do you feel to see something besides bills and junk mail?

While you read the letter, the handwriting of the person who cared enough to write reminds you that wherever that person was a few days ago, whatever was going on in her life, she thought it was worthwhile to pause long enough to write you a letter.

That's how I felt when I received a letter from a friend named Anne, one month before my first baby was due. She had taken the time to fill an entire page with bullet points that featured advice and encouragement for the postpartum journey to come. It was written in her own beautifully artistic handwriting, just for me.

Those first few weeks of managing a newborn, I turned back to Anne's letter often. During that time in my life when so many things were changing, her handwritten notes helped me feel normal. They helped me remember I was not alone as I navigated the ups and downs of my postpartum world.

Anne's notes to me were so meaningful that I began to write my own list of bullet points like hers—advice for other friends who were about to have their first babies. My hope was that they might benefit from them the way I had.

One day I got a call from Bri, my former college roommate, who lived across the country. Our conversation lasted about five seconds before she blurted out, "I'm pregnant!" She literally could not contain herself, she was so happy. This was her dream, and although it happened a little later in life than she planned, it was finally her turn. She was over-the-moon excited as she drilled me with questions. Like an exuberant little sponge, she wanted to soak up as much insight as possible about what to expect as she headed into these uncharted waters.

This girl needed more than one page of bullet points!

And so, I wrote her an entire letter. And then I wrote eight more. I sent one at the beginning of each new month of her pregnancy, finally concluding when she was in the hospital with her brand new baby boy. Bri, the sweet, wonderful soul that she is, expressed such happiness after receiving these letters. She encouraged me to compile them into a book for other pregnant mamas to enjoy.

So kick back, relax, and have fun reading! I hope you find these letters personal, my friend. I hope they make you feel like the beautiful, radiant, empowered pregnant mama that you are. I hope they make you feel loved, encouraged, and more prepared. Most of all, I hope they make you feel blessed by our amazing God.

hallelujah!

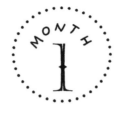

Happy Unpleasantries

My dear friend,

PRAISE JESUS! HALLELUJAH! YOU'RE HAV-
ing a baby! Your time is finally here! It's your
turn to embrace the crazy beautiful chaos that is
pregnancy and motherhood. Rest assured; God has
given you everything you need to take it on!

I have so many questions for you.

How did you find out?

How did it feel, the moment you knew for sure?

How did your husband find out? Are you still waiting to find the most amazing way to tell him?

Have you told anyone else, or am I the special number one?

How long have you been praying for this? Did God surprise you with a plan different than your own?

Even if you don't keep a journal or consider yourself a writer, I encourage you to write down the thoughts and feelings churning inside you during this special and unique time in your life. The answers to your questions above are fresh in your memory now, and I'm guessing they are precious enough that you'll never want the details to fade. There will be so many opportunities for reflection in the coming months. Writing them down as you have the time (even just one or two sentences) is a great way to cement them in your memory so you can look back on them down the road.

This is a big deal, my friend. You're having a *baby*!

How are you feeling?

Pregnancy stirs up a lot of new ingredients in the recipe of you. You'll experience a mix of emotions that you've never felt all at the same time: joy, fear, excitement, gratitude, worry, trust, doubt, and a little bit of terror. This can make you feel a tad overwhelmed at times.

Now add in the countless anecdotes you've heard and will continue to hear over the next nine months about how others' pregnancies have gone, and you might start to form certain expectations about what's going to happen to you.

The thing about pregnancy is that there are a million ways yours could be different from the stories you've heard. This can leave you in a constant state of wondering, "Is this normal?"

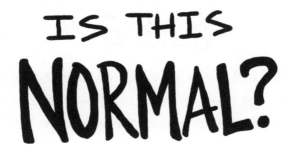

IS THIS NORMAL?

That's why I'm here. Although I can't possibly cover every symptom or scenario you might encounter, my goal is to help you feel confident, encouraged, positive, and...well, normal.

I want to be your personal cheerleader on this nine-month journey to mama-hood.

I've written you a letter for each of the next nine months that features an in-depth analysis of different aspects of pregnancy. These letter are full of candid truths, genuine love, and encouragement. There will be some unsolicited advice and an occasional dose of comic relief. So, without further ado, our first focus:

HAPPY UNPLEASANTRIES

Happy unpleasantries? Happy vomiting? Yes! Although the inconvenient and not-so-lovely symptoms of early pregnancy can make you feel less than stellar, they are telling you that your baby is still going strong in there! Feel free to moan and groan while you're hugging the toilet bowl before

you head to work in
the morning. Deep
down, do your happy
dance, and use it as
a reminder to thank
God for this pregnancy.
After all, you did ask for this, right? Did
you? I can't remember.

Before I go any further, know that not everyone
has the hallmark discomforts of early pregnancy. In
other words, don't panic if you *aren't* experiencing
morning sickness. Its presence is a nice reassurance that you are, in fact, pregnant, but its absence
doesn't necessarily mean something is going wrong.
You could very well be blessed with a body that is
perfectly content being pregnant.

If not, here are some tips for persevering through
those happy unpleasantries:

Nausea

Avoid long boat rides on windy seas, if possible.

I realize this one is rather unlikely, but it reminds
me of a story you might enjoy. My husband, Phil,
and I visited Dry Tortugas National Park when I
was six weeks pregnant. If you're unfamiliar with

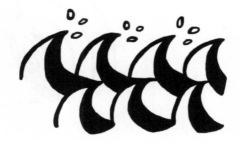

it, this park is a small island fort 70 miles off the coast of the Florida Keys. To get there requires a 2-hour and 15-minute ferry ride. The wind was fierce that day, and the waves were three to six feet high. I spent the majority of the trip on the back deck holding a barf bag with my eyes fixed on the horizon, because the guy working his first-ever shift on the ferry (also struggling not to throw up) told me it might help. It did help a little; I only lost my cookies once! And then, of course, at the end of the day, we had to ride the nausea ferry back to the mainland. I couldn't handle eating anything until breakfast the next day when my feet had been on solid ground for a good 15 hours. This was miserable. I recommend waiting until you aren't pregnant to tackle long sea excursions.

Keep bland crackers in a drawer at work and by your bedside. I recommend something like saltines, oyster crackers, or multigrain crackers with no seasoning except salt. When the nausea hits, start nibbling.

It's possible for the aroma of peppermint to calm the tummy as well. During pregnancy, however, it might be a toss-up because you could also be extra sensitive to smells. It might be worth a try to chew a stick of peppermint gum, knowing it's a trial-and-error tactic. If it doesn't work for you, at least you tried. (Please don't come after me if it turns you off to the flavor of peppermint for life. I'm sorry!)

If you can, keep a trash can close by for peace of mind.

I also found car sickness to be an issue in my pregnancies. When you are a passenger, admire the scenery instead of scrolling on your phone or reading a book. Obviously, it's best to avoid these things if you're the driver, too. Not only will it help with car sickness, but also with your likelihood of surviving the drive. You have extra precious cargo now. Think twice before glancing away from the road. It's not worth the risk.

Vomiting

Keep a toothbrush, toothpaste, and breath mints in your purse. There's nothing like rejoining your clients or coworkers with barf breath.

It's also a good idea to keep your toilets really clean. It will make morning sickness (which doesn't always abide by the confines of morning, by the way) just a teensy bit less awful.

Some lucky ladies don't throw up at all; some just a few times; some like clockwork. Once in a while, a poor woman can have this symp-tom so badly that she can't eat and begins to lose weight at an unhealthy level. I pray this doesn't happen to you, friend! But if it does, tell your doctor right away so he or she can help you keep that baby safe and strong.

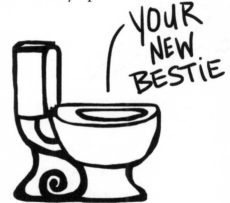

YOUR NEW BESTIE

Bloating and Constipation

Sometimes you'll look down and think, "Oh man, here comes the bump!" Then, perhaps you'll realize that you're just that bloated. Not exactly the moment to make you feel like a beautiful, radiant, expecting mama, is it? You may feel *so full* inside—which makes sense, of course, given the fact there's a human growing in your uterus. From now until delivery, your bladder, uterus, intestines, stomach, and liver will be fighting for prime position in your abdomen, but the uterus will always win. It's natural for your other functions to feel a bit backed up.

For a jolly good time, look up a YouTube video about where all your organs go during this process. It's a little freaky, but it explains so many of the digestive symptoms you may have in the later months of your pregnancy.

Speaking of the digestive system, eat lots of high fiber foods. Fruit, dark-colored vegetables, and everyone's greatest temptation: bran! Metamucil (a fiber supplement—not to be confused with a laxative!) was my friend during the postpartum

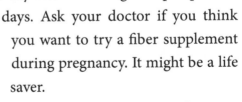

days. Ask your doctor if you think you want to try a fiber supplement during pregnancy. It might be a life saver.

Drink a *lot* of water! This may intensify your urge to urinate, but you will feel so much better. Water will help keep things moving through your system, decrease headaches, and give your baby the hydration he or she needs.

If you're like me and have trouble remembering to drink water, set alarms on your phone for times during the day you know you can drink a glass or refill your bottle. You can also set daily or hourly ounce intake goals. One useful tool that exists for this purpose is a special water bottle with different times of the day descending down the side. This will help you visualize how much you should drink by 10 a.m., noon, 2 p.m., etc. You can find them online, and they cost about the same as a typical big water bottle.

Did I mention you should drink more water and that fiber is your friend? Water…fiber…keep things moving! If you do end up with a traffic jam, prune juice may be an effective solution.

Sore Boobs

There's not a whole lot you can do about this one. You are literally growing new duct work in there that didn't exist before.

If this becomes a severe problem for you, try ice packs. Believe it or not, there are ice packs that come in the shape of boobs. A light heating pad can also help, as can kindly reminding your husband that your boobs are quite sore if he starts getting handsy.

Bathroom Surprises

It's wise to keep a couple panty liners stashed in your purse throughout your pregnancy. There are several things that could catch you off guard at inconvenient times: spotting (a little early on can be normal, but anything significant warrants a call to your OB, which I'm sure you've been told), mucus-like discharge, and, unfortunately, urine.

I wish I could say I never peed myself while pregnant, but I can't. Picture being on a boat in late summer two weeks before your due date (here we go again, back on a stupid boat). You're laughing and having a grand ol' time, only to find out upon standing up that your water has broken. Hooray! Time to have a baby! Oh wait... false alarm. You just peed yourself with- out even knowing

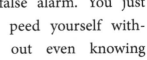

it…in front of your husband's parents, sister and extended family. And there was no one who *didn't* see it. Glorious. It happens. Everyone will still love you!

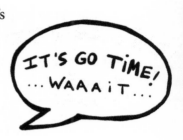

But, to bring these points home on a happy note, rejoice in the knowledge that you won't have your period for nine months!

TRUSTING THE CREATOR

Before I end my letter for this month, I want to touch on something that has no doubt crossed your mind by this point—something more serious than seasickness and bathroom quandaries. At this early stage of pregnancy, the chance of loss is unspoken, but on the mind.

I'm sure you've heard stories from friends or family members who have endured miscarriages. My friend, I pray you have never experienced this yourself. It's okay to be scared about this possibility. Of course it is.

But do not let the possibility cripple you.

Instead, use it as an opportunity to give God the wheel.

Any life, at any moment, may end. That's the reality we live with every single day, and every so often we see this direct result of sin rear its ugly head. A ride in the car, a fall down some steps, a silent clot in the vessels of the brain. There are so many ways humankind is breakable.

The response to these fears is simple: Trust that God is in control and working for your good—even when the inevitable consequences of sin surround you. Notice, I said "simple," not "easy." This response doesn't come naturally to the sinful human flesh, which yearns to be in control. Yet, grace is bigger than fear. Jesus has washed you clean, made you His, and given you a reason not to fear.

Trusting God with your baby's life begins now at this early stage of pregnancy. It will continue throughout the baby's life, however long that is. We hope and pray that the earthly life of each new baby

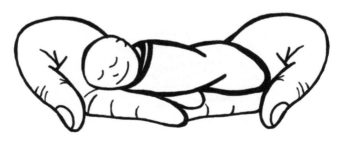

is long, healthy, and happy. As believers, we can find tremendous peace in God's promises, knowing that he is compassionate and "showing love to a thousand generations of those who love me and keep my commandments." (Exodus 20:6)

This sin-stained earth is not our home. Heaven is.

Giving God the wheel means trusting that He wants your babies in heaven. Whether they arrive sooner or later, it's part of God's brilliant and inconceivable plan, just as it was when He knit them together inside you. Whatever that plan is, have peace knowing that He will never abandon you or your new baby.

Allow yourself to be happy and confident in God's plan for your child. Be thankful for every moment of your pregnancy, even the seasickness and bathroom quandaries.

Don't be afraid to tell close family or friends about your pregnancy already. Ask them to pray for you and

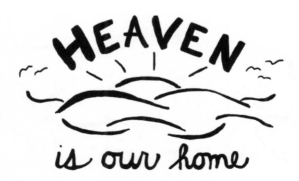

your little one! They are your support team in the good and the bad, and it will only be a blessing to have them on your prayer force in any situation.

My friend, have fun being pregnant! There is nothing else like it. It's your turn to glow and dream and love like never before. God is watching over you, holding you and your baby in his hands. He's promised to bless you in so many ways—most importantly, with grace and peace in this miracle called life and with the sure hope of heaven beyond.

> "Do not worry about anything, but in everything, by prayer and petition, with thanksgiving, let your requests be made known to God. And the peace of God, which surpasses all understanding, will guard your hearts and your minds in Christ Jesus."
>
> —Philippians 4:6-7

You're going to rock this, you beautiful girl!

Love, Kristen

P.S. Remember to grab a journal and start scribbling some memories. You'll be so glad you did!

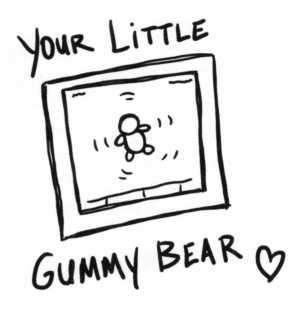

YOUR LITTLE

GUMMY BEAR ♡

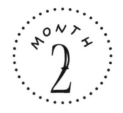

Body Image

My dear friend,

YOU'VE SEEN AN ULTRASOUND IMAGE OF your baby on the screen. You have a printout of your little eight-week-old miracle blob.

Side note: Does it bother you they count the first two weeks before conception in the estimated age of your child? You weren't even pregnant yet, so why include them? Why don't they subtract two weeks from your last period for a more accurate age? If that bothers you like it does me, let's secretly acknowledge that your blob child is really only six weeks old, making the speed of development that much more astounding! Okay, moving on…

Now it's real. You have proof, beyond a doubt, that there is a human growing inside you. Totally and completely mind-blowing. And what's more, your baby keeps growing—every minute, every second—without you even thinking about it or helping it along. Well, besides drinking water instead of alcohol and avoiding excessive amounts of donuts, of course. *Amazing.*

God has designed your body to do truly remarkable things. You should be so proud of that beautiful masterpiece!

That's what your body is, my friend—a beautiful masterpiece.

It's so easy during pregnancy and postpartum healing to feel like you've changed rapidly from hot babe to hot mess. Therefore, before we go any further, let's address the topic of:

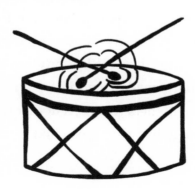

BODY IMAGE

Cherish the Bump

It's natural to fear the bump at first. After all, it's a bit weird. You especially might be dreading that awkward phase when your tummy is just starting to look bigger than has ever been normal for you. Others might think you just overate Thanksgiving dinner or put on several pounds of marriage pudge. Makes you feel sexy, right?

Don't worry, friend. Trust me when I say that you are your own worst critic. Be confident in your body and the way God is working miracles through it. Chances are, no one notices these changes like you do.

Despite its weirdness, the bump has advantages. As it grows, it becomes an unmistakable sign to the outside world that A) you could use some help lifting heavy things at the store, and B) there is a second life inside you. Be proud! Savor this short-lived and unique feeling. It's a constant, visual reminder of baby's progress and the only physical barrier between your loving hands and that precious little mystery within.

I won't deny that the bump will start to feel cumbersome by the last few months of your pregnancy. Turning over in bed, lying down in bed, getting out of bed, getting comfortable in bed, being intimate with your husband in bed…pretty much any activity relating to your bed will be very difficult. Not to mention tying your shoes, walking long distances, and prolonged standing or sitting. Maybe you'll be lucky enough to be repeatedly kicked in your sciatic nerve. Needless to say, it will feel pretty good to eventually get rid of the you're-about-to-pop-sized bump after the full nine months. It will be bittersweet though. You might occasionally miss that

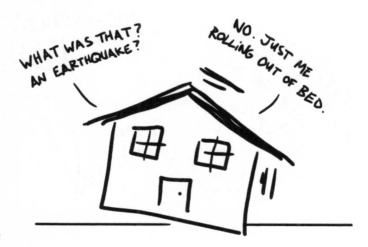

indescribable closeness that no one else can experience besides you and your baby. So try to laugh about these things and just savor, savor, savor.

In regards to staying as comfortable as possible in bed, I recommend using a long body pillow or one of those fancy pregnancy pillows if you're feeling wild. Since sleeping on your side is really the only position you'll be able to use for several months, lying with the body pillow under your top arm, wedged between your belly and the bed and between your knees and ankles will keep your belly supported and your spine in a happier alignment. It will help you sleep more comfortably and avoid back pain.

When it comes to feeling good about your new look during the day, my advice is simple. Have fun! We are so blessed in today's world to have many styles of maternity clothes to choose from. You can wear flowy tops that conceal the bump during the faux-marriage-pudge stage or tighter fitting tops that make it a little more obvious you have a baby bump. Take your mom, your husband, or a friend to your local maternity store and have a blast trying out new looks.

Warning! This can get pricey. Here are some ideas for keeping the receipts a little smaller:

Start at the clearance racks. Maternity stores have them, just like most other stores.

Department stores like Target and Walmart may have small maternity sections. Call ahead to make sure you're not wasting your time looking there, since not all locations have them.

Ask recently-pregnant friends or family if you can borrow their maternity clothes (and of course, make sure to give them back when you're done). Since maternity clothes are only worn for a few months at a time, you can get a nice little exchange going where you trade your clothes back and forth with each new pregnancy in the group.

Scour thrift stores. Again, since maternity clothes are not typically used that long, you can find some great like-new apparel at your local thrift store for a fraction of the cost of buying new.

Tiger Stripes

You can do your best to avoid stretch marks by rubbing Vitamin E oil, lavender oil, coconut oil, or anything that helps to boost the elasticity of your skin over problem areas like belly, hips, breasts, and love handles. I suggest doing this every day for the most benefit.

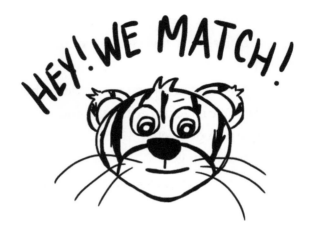

If, after all these preventative measures, you are still graced with stretch marks, call them tiger stripes instead. They are a personal reminder, in a pattern unique to you, of the amazing things God allowed your body to do for this baby. They are a sign of sacrifice, selflessness, and courage. You got this, mama tiger!

Boobs...Just...WOW

Big boobs can be awesome if you aren't accustomed to them. Enjoy! You're welcome, husband.

The local maternity store will once again be your friend. Buying new bras is tricky business. Everyone is so different. You could grow any number of sizes by the time baby gets here. Remember, they will peak in size during the first few weeks after your baby is born. By then, they will have turned into actual milk machines, so you'll have to make your best guess at what you'll need a few weeks before your due date. We'll tackle the treat of engorgement in the postpartum prep letter. Until then, just know your boobs will be huge.

I recommend getting maternity bras that also double as nursing bras. These are designed to be used during pregnancy, but also for breastfeeding once your baby is born. My maternity/nursing bras were super comfy. Honestly, I was bummed when I was done breastfeeding and couldn't fit into them anymore (oh, *so* far from fitting into them anymore). Here are my recommendations:

+ Sleep bras. Get something lacy that makes you feel lovely. Secretly, they are stretchy (to pull down each side for breastfeeding) and totally comfortable for sleeping.
+ Clip-down T-shirt bras that don't have underwire. These are perfect for wearing around the house or at the grocery store. You know, places you don't need to dress up for but still want to look presentable.
+ Underwire clip-down bras that offer full

coverage and give more shape. These will help you feel a little more put together when you venture into public again after the baby is born.

+ Clip-down sports bras. Use these if you plan to do a fair amount of exercising while you're still breastfeeding.

There's one last thing I want to share on this oh-so-intimate topic. One of the least dignifying body changes that got to me during pregnancy and postpartum was leaky boobs. I'll never forget the day I realized, at 20 weeks pregnant, that it would be in my best interest to wear washable or disposable pads on the inside of my bras for the next six to nine months. Ugh. This was one of those things that kept my husband gazing at me perplexedly time and time again, muttering, "Pregnancy is so weird." True. That.

So, I recommend getting some washable bra pads. Pregnancy colostrum is pretty minor (that nutritious yellow stuff you start producing long before the actual milk comes in), but you'll probably want some pads with real absorbency later. Now, before you go crazy stocking up on these little lifesavers, know that the exact severity of leakage varies from person to person. You may want to start with two or three pairs, then upgrade to more if it becomes a bigger issue once the baby is born.

WEIGHT GAIN

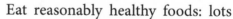

This is the one time in your life when everyone is supportive of significant weight gain (25-35 pounds, anyway). It's a very good thing. Don't let the rising number on the scale freak you out. You can't have a healthy baby without it!

On the other hand, this is *not* an excuse to constantly feast on things that aren't good for you. Eat reasonably healthy foods: lots of fruits and veggies, protein, healthy fats, whole grains, etc. Remember, you only need about 500 extra calories per day, so you're not exactly "eating for two" in the true sense of the term. However, it's not necessary

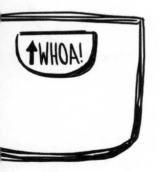

to deprive yourself of all things delicious either. If you crave ice cream, have some ice cream, and don't feel bad about it! It's not going to hurt the baby. Just know where to draw the line if you feel the temptation to frequently overindulge.

As you gain weight, you may notice extra curves in a lot of different places. It's okay, and it has to happen. As long as you are staying moderately active and eating reasonably healthy, these new contours are out of your hands. Embrace the way your body is supporting another human life, and try to find humor in your temporary new look. Most importantly, trust God's process!

On that note, don't fret too much about those abdominal muscles. Believe it or not, they can realign and regain strength again. There are steps you can take in the early postpartum period to help them along.

(You can find a free, downloadable PDF titled *Postpartum Exercise Program* on my website at www.kristenemilybehl.com.) For now, just marvel at how much they can stretch and move to make way for a baby—along with the other contents of your abdominal cavity.

Lastly, although swollen ankles may not actually contribute much to your overall weight gain, they'll sure make you feel like a bloated balloon. God has given us knee-high compression socks to help us deflate, so don't feel like a dork for using them. Own them, mama. Rock those stockings!

THE VOICES AROUND YOU

Never in your life will you hear more comments about your appearance from friends, family, and strangers than when you're pregnant. Some might be uplifting: "You look amazing! That's the cutest little bump I've ever seen!" The next might be the polar opposite: "Oh my goodness, you're not due till September? I didn't think you could get any bigger!" Or my personal favorite, "Don't lean on anything sharp!" Sometimes these starkly different comments will all be made to you in the same day!

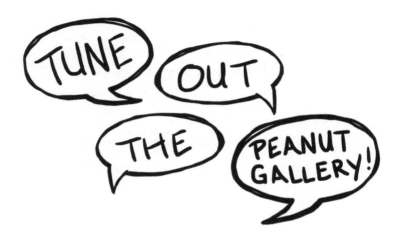

It's unreal, like the presence of a baby bump automatically gives everyone around you permission to comment about your appearance without being offensive. Wrong!

If you progress through your pregnancy feeling self-confident about your appearance, you probably won't get too upset by insensitive comments, and you'll still be grateful for those uplifting comments. On the other hand, if you find yourself struggling with your own appearance as your body changes throughout pregnancy, some comments can feel awfully cruel.

The thing is, no one makes comments like these with malicious intent. You're pregnant, and since this gives you a valid excuse for having extra curves and extra weight, they simply assume it doesn't bother you to hear about it. To them, it's just a conversation piece, a way to connect with you and share a laugh. They don't realize you might not think it's funny, or that it might actually hurt. They don't realize you could have been looking in the mirror earlier that morning worrying about your body.

Frankly, a lot of people don't always think before they speak.

Although you'd rather not fly off the handle at comments from your well-intentioned grandma, I think it's within your right to say something if you want. Usually, if the people who say silly things had any inkling that their comments would bother you, they never would have said them.

So do your best to wrangle the raging tiger inside, and respond kindly with something like, "I'm actually having a hard time with it," or even a simple, "Thank you." Those simple phrases might be enough to help somebody realize a comment was unnecessary or off-color. It will help lead the conversation in a more encouraging direction.

If you prefer to be less confrontational, you could uplift yourself by saying something like, "Yup, my baby is growing healthy and strong in there," or, "God can do some pretty amazing things, don't you think?" This would show the person you'd like to focus on more positive things, and hopefully point the exchange in a better direction.

Unfortunately, there will be folks who still won't get the message. You'll almost certainly encounter at least one relentless Negative Nancy, who, no matter how sweetly you try to change the conversation, will say something like this:

+ Negative Nancy: "Wow, I never thought you would get this big!"
+ You: "Well, I'm trying to focus on the health of the baby, because I tend to worry about how I look even though I can't help it."
+ Negative Nancy: "I'd say that baby must be pretty healthy. You might have to stop feeding him so you don't pop, and you've still got a long way to go!"

Seriously, some people are clueless. It fits right along with that idea that you and your feelings play second-fiddle to baby now. People tend to forget that you are still your own person.

My best advice is to immerse yourself with positive influences—friends, family, husband—people you can rely on to build you up and remind you of the depth of your beauty. Don't shrug it off when someone tells you that you're looking radiant. Soak it up and dwell on it; fall asleep that night with a smile of satisfaction! Let confidence grow inside you, so that when you do receive those off-putting comments, your self-worth will burst through and overpower them like a vibrant flower that breaks through a crack in the sidewalk.

Regardless of how you prefer to respond to the comments, remember that in the grand scheme of things they are trivial. They might be well-intentioned but poorly constructed. Focus on the things you *can* control, not the things you can't. You can't totally control how your body will look. You can't control what the people around you say about it. You *can* control what *you* say about it.

THE VOICE WITHIN YOU

Tell me I'm not the only one. Do you have it too? That voice that tells you these changes you see in the mirror are anything less than beautiful? The voice that subtracts joy from your moment by taunting you, *"You're never going to be the same. You'll never look as good as you did before you had this baby."*

The voice is real, and it's cruel.

It comes partly from the piece of you that genuinely fears the physical changes. Don't beat yourself up for that. Don't deny the feeling. It's normal to have that fear. Your body, as you've always known it, is changing very suddenly...a lot. You don't know exactly what it will be like after you have the baby. It's a scary thing! Acknowledge it to your Creator. Spill your worries to Him in prayer. Tell Him about the fears you have for your body, however legitimate, trivial, or selfish they may make you feel to say them out loud. He already knows you have them, so it's no use trying to hide them from Him. Instead, go to Him for comfort. Let Him hear you.

Ask for His help to achieve the outcome you want. Then ask for peace no matter the outcome. Ask for self-love that transcends concern for outward appearance. You'll be amazed at the things He will do to reassure you.

The other contributor to that nasty voice in your head is the influence of our society that is obsessed with body image. The same barrage of advertisements, photoshopped actresses, and perfectly staged social media photos that make teenage girls self-conscious are continuously being fed to our subconscious minds as adults. It's one thing to take care of the body God gave you and to feel your best—that is a good thing. However, once you notice your self-esteem trending downward in the midst of the physical changes of pregnancy, you are falling prey to the voice. You are falling prey to the lies.

Hear this instead. Your worth is greater than your temporary shell. God's purpose for you on this earth stretches far beyond the confines of your imperfect physical body. Your world is about to get a lot bigger the moment you hold your own sweet child in your arms. There will be times while raising that child that you will stew over all the challenges, including any lasting changes to your body. Far more often, there will be moments that remind you that it's all worth it. Watching your child pray at the dinner table or at bedtime, listening to that little voice sing to Jesus in the back seat of the car, or crumbling when you hear, "I forgive you, Mommy." These things matter more than fitting into that old bathing suit, don't they? If you had to choose between the two, is it even close?

Don't get me wrong—you very well might still fit into that old bathing suit after a while. Even if you don't, despite valiant, healthy human efforts, God's plan is God's plan. He made you beautiful pre-baby, and He'll keep you beautiful post-baby. He made you magnificent inside and out. Everyone else can see that. Can you?

When my two-year-old daughter looks in the mirror, I tell her, "You are so pretty—on the outside and the inside. Do you know what it means to be pretty on the inside?"

She listens, grinning at herself bashfully in her toddler-sized mirror. "Jesus in my heart," she says, touching her little chest. Think of yourself as that precious little girl looking in the mirror. Just because you're a grown up doesn't make it any less true. I want my daughter to remember those words through every stage of her life, and I pray she'll never lose sight of her inner beauty, no matter what the passing time of this earthly life does to her earthly body.

I want the same for you, my beautiful friend. Think of yourself as you see your child—as your mama saw you. Trust that God is taking care of your physical body, and do your best to treat it well. Never lose sight of the bigger picture that your body is temporary, but your soul is eternal. Tell that voice in your head to move aside. You've got a Jesus party going on in your heart, and downers aren't allowed!

Although the nine months of pregnancy are not always flattering, I hope you feel like the exquisite work of art that you are during every moment of it. God literally designed your body for this process.

During pregnancy, you will make people smile just by entering a room. You will make people ponder the beauty and miracle of life without even talking to them. After all this, your body will likely not look or feel exactly like it did before, but it will be worth it. Really, it will!

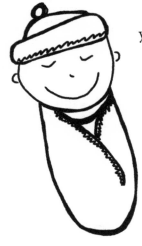

The most important change is that you will have a warm, cuddly, baby-scented child of God in your arms. That's what others see as well. They see the product of love between you and your husband. They see the amazing journey you went through to grow that little miracle. They see the selfless love of a mama radiating from that big beautiful smile of yours.

God is taking care of you and your body, just like He is taking care of baby's. Trust His process.

You are one lovely lady, sweet pregnant mama!

Love, Kristen

"So God created mankind in his own image, in the image of God he created him; male and female he created them."

—Genesis 1:27

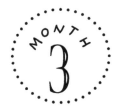

Energy

My dear friend,

CONGRATULATIONS! ANOTHER MONTH OF growth and development for that little baby of yours! You are officially approaching the second trimester. Woot woot! Hooray! Thank you, Jesus, for getting us here!

This is typically the stage when you feel pretty good. Hopefully, any morning sickness you've been experiencing is finally gone, and your cute little bump isn't big enough to keep you from doing the everyday things you enjoy. (Except for drinking wine. Grrrrr! It's a good thing these babies are so adorable.) You should still be able to move around pretty well and feel more energized overall.

Now, before we dive into the great things you can do during this energetic phase, I want to put your mind at ease in case you're feeling less than your usual spunky self. During pregnancy, energy is an anomaly that shifts like the wind. One day you're ready to take on the world, and the next day you feel like a cavewoman dragging your knuckles behind you out of sheer exhaustion. Sometimes you may experience this reversal within the same day.

In this letter, I'm going to cover both ends of the spectrum. Although the second trimester is *supposed* to feel lively, that doesn't mean you won't have moments—even days—of tiredness to remind

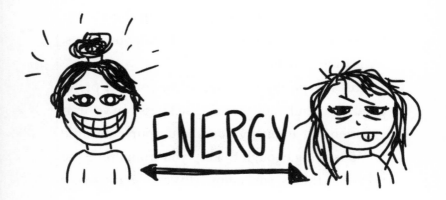

you that you're supporting two lives instead of one. I want to equip you with insights to help you maximize your pre-baby vitality and function through the droopy eyelid periods as well.

INSOMNIA AND FATIGUE

Insomnia, or the inability to sleep at night, is a common symptom of pregnancy. (Don't you worry—once baby comes you shouldn't have trouble falling asleep.) Fatigue, of course, will afflict you while you're pregnant and in the postpartum days that follow.

I'm sure you've heard all the warnings from everyone and their mother about how little sleep you're going to get (as if you don't already know). Maybe you're feeling just a little nervous about that. Maybe you're really freaking out about that. Maybe you're not concerned at all because you know God will help you through it. Maybe you're feeling all three.

Trust me, friend—you can get through this, and God *will* help you!

If you've never had recurring insomnia before, this may be an intense and frustrating new experience for you. It's hard to find joy when you're lying in bed on a work night with your eyes wide open, feeling so tired but not able to sleep, watching the clock tick closer to the start of a long new day.

Take heart! God is smart. He's getting your body ready to function with less sleep to prepare you for life with a newborn. When you're lying there in the middle of the night, instead of being super annoyed that you can't sleep, say, "Thanks for the training, God!"

Here are some ideas that may help you fall asleep and stay asleep:

+ Rub a few drops of high-quality lavender oil on your chest or neck. (You should be able to smell its potency when you hold the open bottle up to your nose.) Or, diffuse the oil in your bedroom right before bedtime. Lavender has been shown to be a great natural sleep aid.

+ Have some quiet time before bed—no TV, no phone. Just read your Bible or another book, write in a journal, or try any other relaxing activity you can do with low light and minimal sound to get your brain ready for sleep.

+ Stretch your calves before you go to bed. (Try searching online if you aren't sure how.) This can help prevent those horrible leg cramps that wake you up whimpering in the middle of the night. Pregnancy is weird.

+ This may sound silly, but have sex! Sharing that time and physical affection with your husband will put both of you in a better mood. It will help you think positively about each other and the baby, and it will increase immediate feelings of happiness and contentment. The happier and more content you feel, the less burdened your mind will be, and the easier you'll be able to sleep. Also, making time and mustering the energy for intimacy (sounds glorious, doesn't it?) is important now more than ever, and will be increasingly important once baby comes storming into your marriage. It's okay to choose sleep over sex sometimes, but don't get into that rut or you may find yourselves never having sex.

+ Use the uninterrupted time to talk to God. Just talk and talk and talk to Him. Of course, while you're pregnant, there's a lot to pray about, and He loves to hear from you. Even if you've been praying for so long that all you have left to talk about is the weather, He still wants to hear about it. Don't feel bad if you fall asleep in prayer. Isn't it a good thing to fall asleep with God on your brain?

+ Keep a pad of paper and pen by your bed, or use your phone on the low-light setting and blue light filter. Then, when you're lying there with random thoughts or to-do lists running through your brain and you don't want to forget them, write them down. It will help you get those topics off your mind so you can go back to sleep.

+ I will get to this in more detail in the next letter, but I recommend selecting a Bible verse
  or verses on which you can meditate during
  labor and delivery. Insomniac moments are
  great opportunities to practice meditating
  on your selected verses. You can draw your
  focus to God's words and *really* think about
  what they mean to you. This will also help
  you to start thinking positively about labor
  and delivery.

If you have a mind that tends to worry when it's
supposed to be resting, here's a cute story for you:

I have a friend whose mind wanders down
bunny trails of what-ifs that get her all worked up
in the middle of the night. Her husband teases her
affectionately about this. He
says her brain is filled
with little mice rac-
ing on their wheels
at all times. When
she's having a frazzled
moment, worrying about
way too many things, her
husband tells her, "Let the
mice rest, hon."

Next time you find yourself in a similar situation, say a little prayer, have a little laugh, let the mice rest, and fall asleep.

And now, some tips to help battle fatigue during the day. At this point in pregnancy, this may not be a big issue for you, but eventually it will be all too applicable:

Decide how best to spend the precious energy you have. What is most important? Getting housework done? Getting work done for your job? Be careful not to neglect things that don't always seem urgent. Perhaps your husband needs some of your time and love but is too kind to ask. Perhaps it's *you* who needs some extra attention from yourself. It's

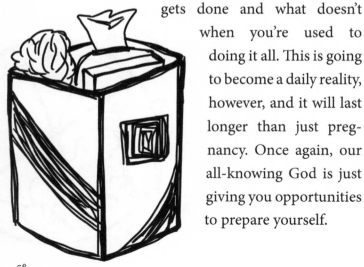

not easy to pick and choose what gets done and what doesn't when you're used to doing it all. This is going to become a daily reality, however, and it will last longer than just pregnancy. Once again, our all-knowing God is just giving you opportunities to prepare yourself.

Know when to ask for help and accept it when offered. If you're 39 weeks pregnant, low on energy, and the cashier at the grocery store asks if you need a carry-out…say yes! This might be hard for you to do because you feel like you *should* be able to do it yourself, or you feel ridiculous getting a carry-out as a young person. Hey girl, listen here! You are pregnant. Everyone adores you. Everyone *wants* to help you. Soak it in. Recognize that this opportunity may never happen again until you're 85 years old, so enjoy it while you can!

Exercise is great during pregnancy for many reasons, but be honest with yourself if your body is telling you to slow down. As your pregnancy progresses, you may find yourself having more shortness of breath, pelvic soreness, even contractions during levels of activity you had no problem with earlier in the pregnancy. Exercise can boost energy, but it can also deplete energy if you overdo it. As you get further along in weeks, consider things like prenatal yoga, aquatic exercise, or brisk walks instead of higher intensity activities. If you're not a gym lover, there are tons of online resources specifically for pregnant women who want to exercise at home.

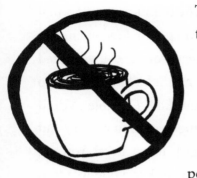

There's something torturous about not being allowed to have much caffeine during this time when you need it most. However, I'm a believer that there's a mental component to caffeine yielding energy. Try to find a replacement (like a power-packed granola bar or nutritious shake powder) that you can turn to when you feel the need for a boost. You'll get the nutrients your body needs to refuel, and mentally you'll still get that shot of energy that keeps you going.

Insomnia and fatigue are two more ways God is telling you to come to Him for rest. Rest in His Word, rest in His peace, and rest in His promises of protection and guidance. These problems can be awfully frustrating in the moment, but do your best to use them to draw nearer to your Heavenly Father. He loves you and that baby even more

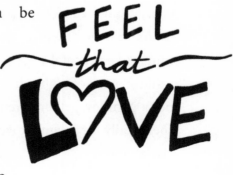

than *you* love that baby. It's unfathomable. Go to Him in these quiet moments and feel that love!

MAKING THE MOST OF THE ENERGY YOU HAVE NOW

All right, enough of that sleepy stuff. Let's talk about the fun you can have in this time of pep and clarity during the second trimester. Yeah, yeah, we all know there are things you can't do while you're pregnant, regardless of how far along you are (alcohol, bounce houses, certainly not the two in combination). Still, there are some wonderful ways to make the most of your time before baby comes in this lovely little window of opportunity.

Travel

I need to preface this one with a disclaimer that your personal ability to travel during pregnancy is just that—personal. It's true that most doctors deem it safe to travel any time before 36 weeks, but if you have some medical complications or anxiety around leaving home during pregnancy, it may not be true for you. Always make sure you check with your physician before you plan a trip.

That being said, if it is safe and desirable for you to travel, put something on the calendar. Most ladies (including me) would tell you that the second trimester is the best time to go. You'll likely have more vigor and fewer physical discomforts during this period. I have taken trips across the U.S. at six weeks, nine weeks, 19 weeks, and 32 weeks of pregnancy. I can say with confidence that 19 weeks was the most enjoyable time to travel. Neither flying nor driving long distances is very easy on the tummy during the peak of the nausea phase, and by 32 weeks the belly just starts getting less comfortable, especially over long distances. However, in that sweet spot of the second trimester, I was able to handle driving and flying, as well as a pretty active itinerary, without any significant issues.

So where should you go? As work schedules allow, try to find something you've been really excited to see or do but haven't gotten around to. You can either splurge and fly somewhere exotic or travel on the cheap

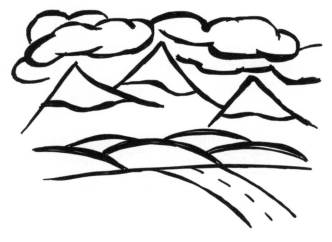

and road trip to a state or national park. Just remember, find someplace that still has plenty of activities appropriate for a pregnant lady! You should also consider local health care in your destination. Make sure you feel comfortable with the available options in the event you would encounter any health issues for you or the baby during your travels.

Ideally, choose something you anticipate will be challenging to do once you have the baby. This is one of your last chances to get away from it all, just you and your husband, for quite a while. It will probably be a few months until you get your feet under you again, and even longer before you'll feel even remotely comfortable leaving baby behind to have an exclusive adventure with your husband. The memories you make together now will be totally worth the scramble it might take to get it organized in the next month or two.

If the budget or PTO don't allow for a big trip, at the very least take a trip out of town together for a weekend. Spend some quality time without distractions. Savor this time just the two of you, while you still have the energy to stay up past nine o'clock. Do what aligns with your own abilities, comfort level, and interests during this time of your pregnancy. Have some fun together!

Socialize with Friends

Well, of course you socialize with friends—that goes without saying. My point is, if you have the choice between online shopping for the baby's crib or going out with friends for dinner, choose going out with friends. It's tempting to get caught up in all things baby, but remember to maximize this opportunity to do the things you might have to put on pause once baby arrives. Have fun with your friends, and savor the freedom.

Date Your Husband

Go to the movies. Go to dinner. Go bowling. Go to a sporting event. Or stay in and cook together and save some money. Have a Packer party for two. (That's right—Go, Pack, Go!) Spend a couple hours being intimate, catching up with each other, talking about the past, the present, and the future.

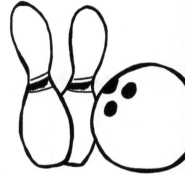

Don't let trivial things interrupt your time together during these dates. Rejuvenating your relationship and prioritizing each other is the whole point. Use this opportunity to refuel your fires. Strengthen your relationship in these months leading up to this major life change, which is inevitably going to make it harder to do things like, say, go on a date. Enjoy the excitement you feel about the days to come, but don't neglect to savor the happiness you find in each other right here, right now.

What if it doesn't feel positively blissful for the two of you right now? What if the stress of the pregnancy and uncertainty of the future are making it hard to feel excitement together? What if there is a disconnect between the two of you because he doesn't seem to understand a lot of what's going on inside your body, heart, and mind?

This sounds like a great reason to go on a

date. Be intentional about it. Communicate with him that you feel this way, and that you want to make it better. Reconnect. Focus your time and energy on each other for the duration of the date. Remember, a strong relation-ship with your husband, centered on Christ's love, is vitally important for parenting this child. It's worth the effort to protect it, to nurture it—because soon, you'll have to lean on it like never before. In a world full of broken families, your child needs parents who demonstrate the love of Christ, not only for the child, but also for each other.

Prioritize this. Do everything you can to com-municate honestly, to listen humbly, and to love, love, love!

Plan...But Not Too Much

Being perfectly mobile and energetic during this phase of pregnancy makes it a great time to get some of that planning done. Sometime in the next three months or so, consider checking the following things off your pre-baby to do list:

+ Make a gift registry. Reach out to friends or mom forums for guidance on what a baby actually needs. New moms can tell you what gems will make your life significantly easier, and what things just cost a lot of money but aren't really worth it.
+ Shop for maternity clothes and nursing tops.
+ Clean out the room you plan to use as a nursery.
+ Design and prepare the nursery.
+ Consider your options and make a decision regarding your employment once baby arrives.
+ Plan and embark on the trip discussed above.

In the end, do not stress out about these things. You have *plenty* of time, little mama. Let these experiences be a blast for you and only add to the positivity and excitement you feel about your new baby. You want to look back on this time with fondness, not as a time when you were pulling your hair out, trying to maximize

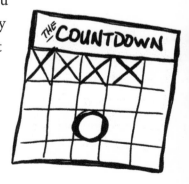

every ounce of energy you had with baby preparations. Your hair will fall out all on its own soon enough (blech, hormones). Don't rush it!

Do What YOU Want To Do

One of the most dramatic changes I noticed after having a baby was losing the ability to simply do what I wanted to do with my time. Of course, even people without children have to go to work when they want to stay home. They have to get up and do the laundry when they'd rather sit and eat ice cream and binge watch their favorite show. It's exponentially more real once you have a baby. When your time is suddenly limited between sleeping, eating, and responding to your baby's every need, it becomes impractical to do what you want. Why? You'll simply have no extra time in which to do it.

It's hard to imagine this level of constraint until you get there, but you'll know what I mean when it happens. Your baby will be worth it, but that doesn't mean there won't be plenty of moments when you'll yearn to have some uninterrupted you-time again.

While you await that precious little life-changer, make sure you enjoy some time doing the things you like to do! Grab that book you've been meaning to

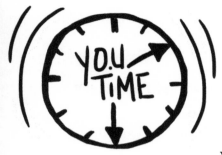

read. Finish that project that's sitting half-done. Go for a hike in places you won't be able to access with a stroller. Nurture whatever hobby you have and enjoy the freedom to do it!

Treasure this phase, dear friend. There will never be a time in your life quite like this, even in subsequent pregnancies. If you are so blessed, the next time around you might have a toddler, and you won't be quite so free to use this second trimester time on yourself, your husband, or your friends.

You have the perfect trifecta of circumstances right now—the excitement of knowing you'll soon have your very own child, the freedom to behave like an adult without kids, and the energy to harness both of these things into positive experiences every day.

Use this gift. Make some great memories!

I pray God blesses you and baby, day after day after

day, sweet friend!

Love, Kristen

"He says, 'Be still, and know that I am God.'"

—Psalm 46:10a

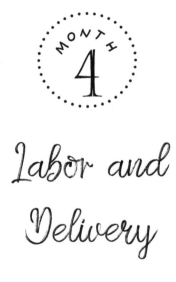

Labor and Delivery

My dear lovely pregnant friend,

ALL RIGHT, SISTER, HERE IT IS—THE LETter you've been waiting for. Even though it's only month four, things are likely starting to feel real enough to make the big day begin creeping toward the forefront of your mind. Since the second trimester tends to leave you feeling symptom-free, what else do you have to think about but the scary, dark cloud looming ahead? Here we go! Let's tackle the big topic:

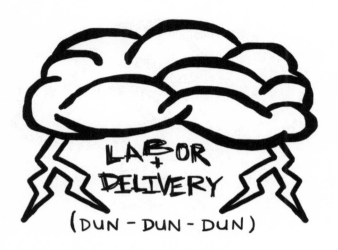

LABOR AND DELIVERY

Before going any further, I'd like to preface this entire section with one simple statement:

Every body is different.

While you are reading this letter, keep the following thought in mind: No two labors and deliveries are exactly the same.

When you're headed to the hospital with your own real contractions, there's nothing you've read or heard that can predict exactly what's about to happen in your story.

When you're finally holding that baby in your arms, reflecting on how your day unfolded, do not compare it to anyone else's.

Your perception of pain is different than anyone else's. Your medical history is different. Your speed of progression will be different. Your medical staff and labor coach will be different than that of your friends.

So many mamas feel disappointed when things don't go according to plan—the plan they've formulated after reading and hearing the experiences of others. It's not fair to do that to yourself! Your story is *your story*. No one else's. God wrote it for *you*.

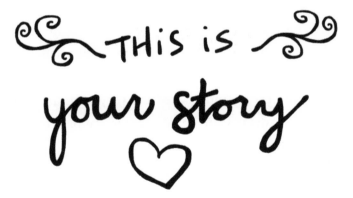

AUTHORED BY: **GOD** (N<u>O</u>T YOU)

You can read all my brilliant insights below, feel totally ready for labor and delivery, and still be baffled to find your experience completely different from what I've described. That's why, although it's

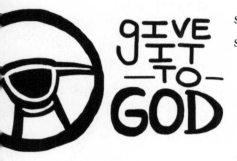 smart to educate yourself on what to expect, your experience with labor and delivery will all boil down to one thing: You have to give God the wheel.

VAGINAL DELIVERY BASICS

You may already be clear on the difference between labor and delivery, but here is a brief description of what the progression might look like—keeping in mind that no one's experience is exactly the same. This is from my personal perspective of a hospital-based delivery with an OB/GYN. The details will be different if you plan to use a midwife or have a home birth.

"Going into labor" refers to having real contractions that come in fairly regular intervals of time. They will increase in frequency and discomfort as time goes on. Don't be deceived by the stereotypical movie scenes where the pregnant lady is fine one second, then suddenly realizes "It's time!" sending everyone around her into a panicked frenzy.

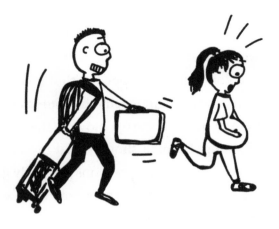

This type of scene might be realistic if your water breaks unexpectedly at home or while you're out and about. While that's a possibility, it's not nearly as likely as a gradual journey through labor when you may be uncertain whether you're actually in labor or not. Of course, that movie scene wouldn't be nearly as exciting, would it?

So, what do real contractions feel like? They can be a little different from person to person, so my description may not be exactly how it feels for you, but it should be close. My contractions woke me up at 3:00 a.m. They felt like a wave of period cramps that originated in my back and wrapped around the front of my lower abdomen. They came and went every 10 minutes or so. They weren't all that intense or painful, just mildly uncomfortable and consistent. It actually had happened the previous night as well, but when I got up and started moving around, the contractions stopped within a couple hours. The following night when it happened again and I got out of bed and started moving, they were still going strong. I took a shower, read my Bible, and made breakfast. The contractions gradually got stronger and closer together. That's how I knew it was go time.

I'd recommend downloading a contraction tracker app on your phone as the due date approaches. That way, when you start feeling those real contractions, you can just push a button on your app to mark the start of the contraction and again when the contraction is over. The app will convert your recordings to a graph showing how far apart your contractions are and how long they are lasting. You can spend your time savoring the experience rather than watching the clock.

That being said, sometimes contraction tracking can become an obsession and make you feel up-tight. If you feel this happening while your contractions are still quite far apart, try to hold off on tracking them until you can tell they are getting close and consistent enough to indicate you may need to head in soon.

Typically the doctor will recommend heading to the hospital when your contractions are one minute long, five minutes apart, for one hour. It might not follow that exact pattern (mine didn't), but you can always call the labor and delivery nurse if you aren't sure whether you should come in. Keep in mind, just because you show up at the hospital doesn't

RULE

5 MINUTES APART
LASTING ABOUT

1 MINUTE LONG
FOR ABOUT

1 HOUR

mean they'll admit you. If they do a triage exam and decide you haven't progressed enough, they can send you home and tell you to come back later. Obviously, that can be annoying, so try to hold out at home as long as possible.

I highly recommend eating something before going to the hospital. Once you are there, they likely won't allow you to eat any solids, in case you end up needing anesthesia. Eat something easy to digest, like bread, soup, fruit, or juice. Some ladies get pretty nauseous (and sometimes even throw up) during labor and delivery, so don't eat anything

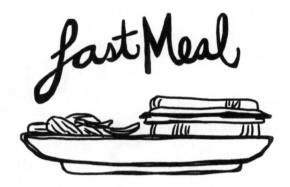

crazy that's going to upset your stomach.

Once you arrive at the hospital, they will place you in a triage room and have you put on a hospital gown. They'll determine how dilated your cervix is, monitor your contractions, and check baby's heart rate to see if you're in true labor. (Heart rate and contractions are seen on a monitor; dilation is a physical assessment your nurse will do with her hand. The invasion of personal space begins!) This is where they can admit you or tell you to go back home for the time being. It's a little nerve-wracking!

Once you are admitted, what happens next will totally depend on your personal scenario and the decisions you make about pain control, etc. If everything is going smoothly and your delivery is considered low-risk, you may only need intermittent monitoring. That means you and your hubby

LAST MATERNITY DRESS!

can walk around the halls, play cards, do some squats, bounce on the stability ball, or do whatever you please to occupy yourselves and help baby along until the contractions intensify enough to keep you in your room. The more you can stay mobile, the better for helping baby's progress. Every so often your nurse will check baby's heart rate and your contractions, as well as your dilation. Your OB will make an appearance somewhere in there as well.

Contractions will gradually intensify, and dilation should gradually increase as the hours go by. These time frames are totally different for each mama. It's possible for dilation to progress very steadily, but it's also possible for dilation to stall for a while. During this time you will decide what to do based on how you're feeling and how much you can still tolerate being up and about. You may need to lie down and rest a bit, which will give you a chance to start zeroing in on your mental hardiness. Somewhere during this time there will be a cutoff for requesting an epidural. Once your contractions get to the point where you can't sit still long enough to administer it, they won't allow you to get one.

My first baby took about eight hours to go from a dilation of 3 cm to 10 cm. Phil and I spent hours walking the halls of the maternity ward. We even stopped by the room next door to visit a friend who had delivered her baby two days earlier and was about to go home. It was a slow but smooth process for the most part. With my second baby, we were in the hospital for less than 90 minutes before she was born. I was already at 7 cm when we were admitted, and everything progressed much faster. It's true what they say: The body tends to know what it's doing the second time around!

Delivery begins only after you reach 10 cm. Not 9 ½ cm…10. There is a risk of swelling that can prevent the baby from being able to come out if you push too early, which can result in a C-section.

The contractions will be quite intense by then, and you will likely start feeling an overwhelming urge to start pushing. (In both of my deliveries, this urge to push started right after my water broke.) As soon as the nurse feels that you are 10 cm dilated, the room will suddenly fill with people. (Up to this point it's only been you and your husband or another support person, along with an occasional visit from your nurse or tech.) They all know their roles to a T. You will go into performance mode. As soon as everyone is in position, you will be free to push in sync with your contractions, and your crowd of cheerleaders will be going nuts with each one. Your husband (or alternate support person) will be right by your side, encouraging you, taking cues from the medical staff on where to stand and how to help you. You probably won't have a super clear vision of what's happening around you at that point. You'll be laser-focused on pushing that baby

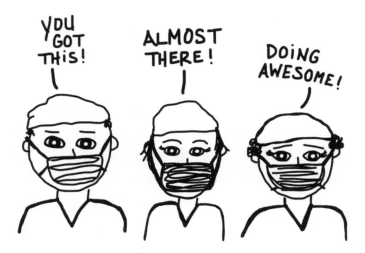

out, catching your breath in between contractions, and taking in the auditory stimuli. No sporting event crowd has ever sounded like that crowd of medical staff and your husband as they cheer you on!

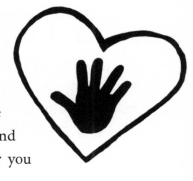

Finally, in a single moment, your baby will be on your chest, and you'll get to see him or her for the very first time. A lot will still be happening to you and around you, but you won't even notice most of it. You'll be too breathless, staring at your beautiful child. Everything else will be background noise. In that moment, it will all be worth it.

CESAREAN SECTIONS

Even though I've never had a C-section, I do want to give you some insight into what that process will look like, just in case you find yourself there. I asked a wonderful friend named Becca to share her experience of a scheduled C-section.

A C-section can be scheduled for the purpose of safety in the event there is something that would cause a vaginal birth to be especially dangerous for mom or baby. A common scenario is when the baby is still in breech position (feet down rather than head down) in the last month of the pregnancy. In Becca's case, they had found an issue with her baby's kidneys that would have made it dangerous for the baby to undergo the trauma of squeezing through the birth canal. Of course, if you have an emergency C-section, much of the prep time will be expedited and the process will look a bit different than Becca's.

LiKE iT OR NOT, I'M COMiNG OUT THiS WAY!

Like most, Becca's surgery was scheduled early in the morning, at 8:00 a.m. She was instructed to arrive two hours beforehand to have the necessary prep work done, so she was at the hospital by 6:00 a.m. She was told not to eat anything that morning, which is hard for a pregnant lady! She stayed up pretty late the night before to eat as late as possible, in order to avoid feeling starved or lightheaded when she went in for surgery.

When Becca arrived, her husband, Tom, got to be in the prep room while nurses asked intake questions. She was then asked to put on a gown, and they shaved her bikini area as the incision is quite low. They took her vitals and did various other preparations for the surgery in that first room.

She then walked to the operating room in her hospital gown. Tom was not allowed in the OR at that point, though policy differs from hospital to hospital. She sat upright on the operating table while a nurse applied electrodes, and the anesthesiologist started prepping her back.

Not a fan of needles to the spine? It's okay. Neither was Becca. She remembers being so nervous during this phase that she was sweating even though it was chilly in the room. Turns out, it didn't hurt at all. She doesn't remember feeling any significant pain or even any pressure as the spinal block was applied. Her feet started feeling numb right away, so they laid her on the table. Of course, with no ability to keep her legs together, she describes this phase with an accepting laugh as "dignity gone!" They put a catheter in, but she didn't feel it at all.

One of the unexpected procedures she recalls was when they strapped both her arms to the table,

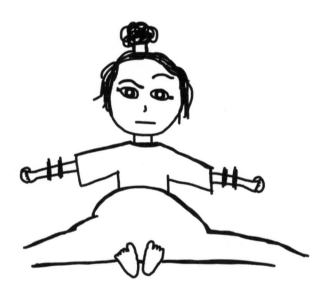

straight out to either side. They do this so you can't accidentally roll off the table, move during the surgery, or grab your baby out of excitement and contaminate the surgical area. It makes sense, really. Since you'll be awake the whole time, there is real potential for dangerous movement.

This seems like it would be a great time to remind yourself to give God the wheel. I can't imagine how it would feel to be strapped down on top and completely

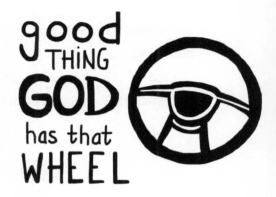

numb and unable to move on the bottom. I guess it might make you feel vulnerable and not in control. It sounds scary, but Becca sends reassurance that although it surprised her, it really didn't make her uncomfortable. She had a lot of adrenaline pumping by that point. And of course, when you know you are going to have a baby within the hour, it helps keep everything in perspective. Trust that your Savior is right there beside you, taking care of you through each and every moment!

Becca also wants you to know that it's okay to feel overwhelmed, and it's okay to cry. Don't let it make you feel ridiculous or weak. The combination of hormones, excitement, and anxiety are not easy to contain, especially when you're numb and strapped down to the table, and your support person isn't in the room with you. The medical staff are typically quite compassionate and will do whatever they can to help you through this experience. Becca's nurse held her hand as she started getting teary, telling her it would be all right. The anesthesiologist called for someone to bring Tom into the room to comfort her. They care about you, new mama! They will help you get through this.

Becca and Tom couldn't actually see the surgery happening, as there was a sheet set up across her chest that obscured their view. I do believe some facilities will use a clear sheet if you really want to watch. The surgeon made the incision at 8:00 a.m., and their daughter was declared born at 8:15 a.m. "It was very efficient," she recalls.

Because of the spinal block, you'll likely feel pressure during the surgery, but not pain. Becca vividly described the sensation: "It felt like someone was grabbing me and pulling me from my stomach. It was weird, like they were pushing pretty hard to get her out." But it was never painful. I do know another mama who had referred pain in her collar bone during her C-section. This just means the pain receptors in the area of the incision are sending signals to the brain, but they are being interpreted as collar bone pain. This phenomenon, called referred pain, is similar to when a heart attack is giving someone the sensation that the left arm hurts. There's nothing wrong with the arm or the collar bone. This doesn't happen for everyone, and it's certainly not the same degree of pain you would feel without the anesthesia, so it's best not to spend time worrying about this. Most likely, you will feel no pain.

After Becca's daughter was born, the nurse cut the umbilical cord, held her up for Becca to see, then brought her to the exam table right away to do the standard APGAR testing. Sometimes babies born via C-section don't cry right away because the mouth and nose are still full of amniotic fluid, having not had time to get rid of them as they would have in the birth canal. Becca's baby did happen to cry right away, but don't worry if yours doesn't. Becca got to hold her baby as soon as they were done with the testing (after her arms were unstrapped, of course).

Keep in mind, these descriptions are based on the experience of one person. Don't panic if yours look a little different when you get there.

The most important thing is to trust in your mighty Protector, who has had your child's delivery day planned since before you were born. So, when some well-meaning lady tells you her horror story, nod politely and reassure her that you trust God's plan for your big day, and that you *know* it will be okay. Tell her you plan to give God the wheel.

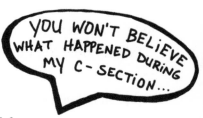

GENERAL TIPS TO PREPARE FOR LABOR AND DELIVERY

Think positive! The first half of my first pregnancy I absolutely *dreaded* the thought of actually giving birth. I was terrified. One day, I finally prayed my heart out about it and placed my fears on God, and I felt so much better from then on. I was able to think positively and expect a smooth delivery, knowing God would protect me and baby and get us through it—and He did! Negative thoughts do not help, so try to nip them in the bud and send them to

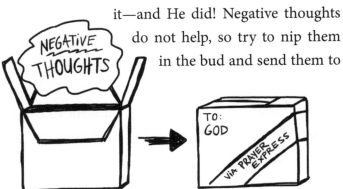

God the moment you feel them coming.

Taking time to develop breathing control and mental clarity is absolutely essential, in my opinion. Find prenatal yoga videos on YouTube, and use them several times a week to practice these vital skills. My go-to videos were by a nice lady named Sarah Beth. They took 10-20 minutes each and were great for gentle stretching, strengthening, and meditating on Bible verses.

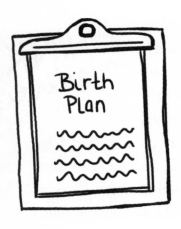

I recommend against a multi-page birth plan for your medical team, spelling out Plans A, B, and C for scenarios X, Y, and Z. If you want to make a birth plan to communicate your desires for your delivery, keep it to one page of the most important things you want them to know. For example, you may want to include whether you want a non-medicated, medicated, or figure-it-out-once-you-get-there delivery, who you plan to have in the delivery room with you, whether you want to delay the Hepatitis B vaccine, things like that. Your nurses may have lots of patients to keep track of, so if you

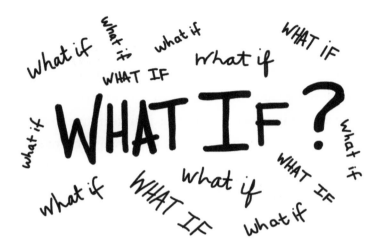

want them to remember anything you write in your plan, it's best to keep it short and sweet.

The truth is, you can spell out a thousand what-ifs, but it could still go differently than expected. It's possible the decisions you'll make when the scenario is actually unfolding are different than you would anticipate on paper. Including a sentence of thanks and trust in your health care team might be a nice touch. I ended up keeping the pain control section of my birth plan to something like this: "I would like to deliver without an epidural, so please avoid offering it. However, if my health or the baby's health requires intervention, I trust you and will be open to your suggestions." And that was it. They never offered it to me, but I'm glad they knew

I'd respect their expertise if they did see a need to change the plan.

There are different schools of thought in regards to allowing labor and delivery to be as natural as possible, as opposed to allowing significant medical intervention. You should make your own decisions about what level of intervention you are okay with, based on the research you have done and what is important to you.

My approach has been to do things as naturally as possible in regards to avoiding heavy medication. However, I welcome interventions that have minimal downsides if they make things significantly faster, easier, or offer protection if things get complicated. For example, with my second baby I was 7 cm dilated when I got to the hospital, but my contractions were slowing down. The doctor told me that she could break my water to stimulate the contractions, rather than waiting to let it happen on its own, which could have taken hours. My husband and I agreed to let my OB intervene by breaking my water. Sure enough, our daughter was born within the hour.

I do know some friends who opted against any unnecessary medical intervention such as this. In the case of one particular friend, her labor lasted several days—but it was important to her, and she is happy that she stuck with her decision. If it's important to you, that's certainly a choice you can make.

Even if you want no other medications, I highly recommend requesting a stool softener or laxative powder like MiraLAX following delivery. It will make that first trip to the bathroom a little less intimidating. At that point you do *not* want to strain your pelvic floor to have a bowel movement. Your nurse or doctor may not automatically offer it, so you might want to write it in your birth plan and be proactive about asking for it.

PAIN CONTROL OPTIONS

Let's delve into pain control options. Remember that whatever route you choose will not result in a trophy either way. There are significant pros and cons to non-medicated delivery as well as having an epidural. Choose what feels right to you and don't feel bad about it!

Non-medicated Pros

+ You can help the baby along by walking and moving throughout most of labor, even once you are admitted to the hospital. Once the contractions are severe enough to keep you in your room, you can still utilize things like stability balls or the tub to help you manage them, rather than being relatively immobile during that time.

+ You can move around and get up sooner after delivery, and you won't have numb legs in the meantime. Also, you won't need a catheter.

+ You can feel if you are pushing efficiently. Believe it or not, there is a right and wrong way to push, and you will be able to feel the difference without the epidural, which can ultimately speed things up.

Non-medicated Cons

+ Obviously, pain is the biggest reason to decide against going non-medicated. As a physical therapist who specializes in pelvic floor rehab, I actually found the sensations kind of fascinating as they were happening (does that make me a nerd?)...but it still hurt. A lot. A lot a lot.

+ As you can imagine, a non-medicated delivery is an extremely intense experience, both mentally and physically. If that's the way you want to do it, I truly believe you can! There is a special beauty in the end result, knowing what it took to get there. However, I want to make sure I express the difference in the whole experience that you'll be opting for. I sometimes wonder if my first delivery would have been a more enjoyable, less traumatic memory if I had chosen the epidural. I mean, I wouldn't change it looking back—but I do wonder...

Medicated Pros (Epidural is most common, but there are other options.)

+ Contractions and pushing should feel more like pressure than pain. Multiple friends have told me they actually didn't mind delivery, and that it was more neat than painful.

+ If you are so tense due to pain that you can't

relax the pelvic floor muscles enough to let progression occur, the epidural has the potential to speed things up.

+ Once again, removing the intense pain of delivery and the mental trauma that may go with it is undoubtedly a huge positive. It can completely change your labor and delivery experience.

Medicated Cons

+ Epidurals can also slow things down for various reasons. For example, you can't help baby along with walking or other movements once the epidural has been administered.

+ For a first delivery, it's harder to know if you are pushing correctly or not, since your sensation is less acute.

+ There is a giant needle getting inserted into the tiny epidural space around your spinal cord. I found this to be more intimidating than dealing with the pain, but I've also heard that it only feels

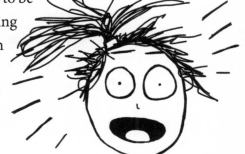

like pressure and is not that painful. Several friends have told me stories that the administration of the epidural did not go perfectly. In one case, it took several tries. In another, it only affected one side, so the woman still felt pain on the other side. In yet another scenario, it caused temporary paralysis in places it shouldn't have. It's not a precise injection, so, unfortunately, those risks exist. However, the majority of people have no problems, so take the anecdotes for what they're worth.

An anesthesiologist in my friend's birthing classes told the students, "You don't *need* me." Remember, God designed your body to be able to give birth! If you want to try a medication-free delivery, know that you can. If you choose not to, have no shame in that. A healthy baby is the most important thing. God also gave us the technology to develop pain medications. Really—it's not cheating to use them.

Tips for Dealing with Pain

Remember how I said mental preparation is vital? I recommend finding a Bible passage that you can memorize and that resonates with you. It should be one that points you to God for strength rather than to yourself. Mine was Psalm 46, especially verse 1: "God is our refuge and strength, an ever-present help in trouble." Start meditating on your verse during your yoga breathing practice. Imagine yourself in labor, using this verse to help you through each contraction. Bring this verse to the forefront of your mind as you consider the pain. Cling to this verse for strength as God guides you through.

Say your verse out loud if you need to during labor. It's a great way to let God shine through you to the medical staff. Let them know where your strength comes from. This may sound odd now, but trust me when I say your normal inhibitions will disappear during labor and delivery. It's a perfect time to evangelize! Make sure your support person knows you plan to use this verse as your mantra, so he or she can help guide your focus there.

When you are having labor pain, particularly

with each contraction, remind yourself of the cause and purpose of the contraction. Each painful contraction means progress! With each one, the baby is getting closer to being out of your body and into your arms. Through your pain, picture your baby dropping down farther and farther.

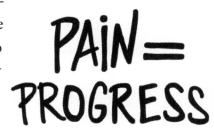

With each push, picture the baby's head getting closer and closer to the outside world. Picture the end goal and how the contractions are helping that goal to be achieved.

Trust your nurses to guide you in alternative pain relief strategies. They know all the tips and tricks, as well as the best times to use them during the labor process. Here are specific strategies I found helpful:

Walking is great early on, when contractions aren't severe. Walk a slow, comfortable pace with your hubby. Laugh, share excitement, and lean on him (literally) when a contraction hits. Savor these last moments together as a couple before that sweet baby arrives. You will never forget this special time with just the two of you.

Sitting on a stability ball or squatting can help

speed dilation, especially if you consciously relax the pelvic floor muscles during these activities. (Think relaxing your muscles like you do to pee.) You can also lean on the stability ball up on the bed. Your body will tell you what position it wants to be in to help manage the pain.

Lying on your side is a great strategy to speed dilation. My nurses suggested it for both my deliveries when one side of the cervix was slow to dilate. Lie on the side you need to dilate more. The nurses will help you figure this out.

If available, the tub makes a great last resort if your contractions are getting severe, but your water hasn't broken yet. (Usually they don't want you to go in the tub if your water has broken due to risk of infection.) You'll get pretty hot in there, so cold cloths for your forehead will help you stay more comfortable. Your nurses will probably be way ahead of you and have all these tips, or more. Seriously, they are amazing.

Aromatherapy is a great option. If your hospital offers it, there are several evidence-based scents that can be beneficial. For example, lavender promotes decreased anxiety and pain; peppermint can be helpful if you are dealing with nausea and vomiting. (Unfortunately this does happen during labor for some).

The Stuff You Don't Want Your Table Mate in the Coffee Shop to See You Reading

Here's a question I bet you never thought you'd ask out loud: How, exactly, do you push out a baby correctly? There are actually some intricacies to consider regarding both positioning and actual technique.

You can deliver in a number of different positions, but most OB's prefer you lying on your back with your knees bent up. Like, way up. Plan on wrapping your arms around your thighs and pushing your legs into your forearms as you try to push the baby out. My biceps were sore for a week!

There are sources that say alternative positions may be better for baby to progress—all fours, side-lying, or even deep squatting, which I can't even imagine. However, my OB preferred the position described above because it was easiest for her to see the baby. It was also easiest for me to save my energy for pushing the baby out instead of supporting my own weight. (The pushing phase will exhaust you quickly, especially if it takes a while.)

With my second delivery, my OB had to stop me from pushing when the baby's head was through, but not the body. She was able to see that the baby's umbilical cord was wrapped around her neck and tightening dangerously as I pushed. She cut the cord from around her neck before delivering the rest of her. My baby did have a delay in breathing, but she eventually took her first breath with the swift help of the NICU doctor in the room. If my OB wouldn't have been able to see that cord entanglement, I wonder if there might have been more serious issues. What I'm trying to say is that I'd rather have the OB use the position of delivery that she is most comfortable with and that allows me to rest between pushes. That's just me. If you do your research and, in collaboration with your physician or midwife, determine that a different position might be better for you, go for it!

And now, let's tackle the actual technique of pushing out a baby. The key—as instructed by my OB after my first few very ineffective attempts—is to "push like you're trying to poop." This is great advice. Seriously, push like you're trying to have the biggest bowel movement of your life. It will be a much more productive push, as that is how our bodies generate the most intra-abdominal pressure. It even helps to hold your breath for a count of 10 while you push, in order to maximize the downward force on the baby by generating lots of pressure in the abdominal cavity.

Please do NOT practice this technique ahead of time. It's not necessary. Aside from delivering a baby, it's not a healthy habit for your pelvic floor to be repeatedly pushed out in this way. Under normal circumstances, you don't want all that pressure forcing things out that are supposed to stay in. (This is how pelvic organ prolapse happens over time.) You should always avoid straining when you use the bathroom so you don't develop this bad habit. But when you're trying to push out a baby, it's a different story. When it's go-time, strain like you've never strained before!

What about the apprehensions you have about embarrassing things that could happen during delivery? Things your dignity doesn't even want to consider a reality?

Let's just lay it out there.

There are a few things that will happen that you wish wouldn't, but there is no avoiding them. They include pooping during delivery, making loud

vocalizations during pushing, being naked in very
strange positions in front of
a lot of people, and making
a very big mess. Most of
these, except the vocalizations, you may not even be aware

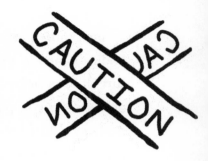

of. You will be so focused on getting that baby out
that none of these absurd things will matter. In
other words, don't worry about these things at all!
They are just every day realities for your medical
team. Your hubs may be surprised, but trust me,
he won't be any less attracted to you. Not even an
ounce. You are his woman, and he loves you more
than anything in the world. All he cares about is
helping you through this miraculous day, holding
his baby, and getting his sex partner back—pronto.

Of note, if you have the epidural, loud vocalizations won't be quite as dramatic. Add that to the
"Pros" column. Let's just say that friend in the room
next door was lucky she left before my actual delivery began. She definitely would have heard me.

Well, that was a fun chat!

Oh wait, I do have one last heads up for you while
we're talking about crazy delivery stuff. After the
baby is born, the nurse will push on your tummy

on several occasions while you're in the hospital. This stimulates the uterus to continue contracting and shrinking, thus preventing hemorrhage—it's kind of super important. Fair warning! It is *shocking* how much this hurts. Seriously, I slapped my nurse as a reflex. Luckily, she didn't seem phased. Did I mention how much I love these nurses?

WHAT TO EXPECT FROM YOUR HUSBAND

Although some husbands are more interested in researching everything there is to know about labor and delivery than their wives are, some aren't. Don't fret if your husband is the latter!

Even though he is not the one going through the physical ordeal, he is the one who has to stand there and watch the love of his life suffer. He has to watch you experience fear and anxiety he can do nothing about. Helpless. That's a very uncomfortable place for a man to be. Not to mention he will be exposed to far more realities of the female condition than he ever has before. We shouldn't hold it against him if he isn't jumping for joy about that.

I got really frustrated with Phil when I started sharing details about postpartum recovery that

I had read about several months before our first child was due. They were quite graphic and he did not respond well to the information. At the time, it made me feel like he wouldn't be ready to be a rock for me in the delivery room. I couldn't have been more wrong! He came through for me in so many ways when I needed him that day. Not only during delivery, but even years later, he still makes me feel beautiful despite the less-than-flattering realities of pregnancy and childbirth. He was so supportive in the delivery room, the nurses told him he could be a doula. Of course, that went straight to his head, and he still shares it with everybody. All right, I do too. I'm so proud of him!

Trust your man. He has anxiety and uncertainty about this day just like you do. Men are different than women. He may prefer to remain blissfully ignorant in the months leading up to go time. He may prefer to take the surprises as they come instead of reading about what's about to happen to his wife. He is your earthly protector, remember, and it's not easy for him to feel helpless, to be unable to lift this burden from you.

Cut him some slack, respect his wishes to know minimal details about what's coming in the delivery room, and trust that he'll be there for you when the time comes. He will beam in your memory as your knight in shining armor, even if all he can do is hold your hand (or your leg) while you push out a baby, offer a word of reassurance in a moment of self-doubt, or make you laugh when you need some comic relief. He will surprise you in so many wonderful ways that neither of you will see coming.

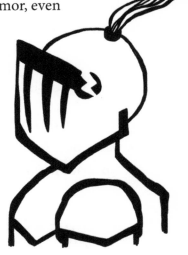

This dynamic is hands-down my favorite part of labor and delivery, even once the baby comes. As I recall the day of my first delivery, I always think of Phil. We laughed together; I leaned on him; he held my hand; he cared for me. Tears welled in his eyes as he saw our daughter for the first time, while his huge hand stroked my hair. It brings me happy tears to this day remembering the love we shared on that snowy Sunday in February.

As much anxiety as you may feel about delivery, let this be your rainbow! Know that you and your man are about to share a bond unlike anything you've experienced before—a bond that is indescribable; one you will never, ever forget.

MATERNITY BAG

What to pack? What to pack? You'll probably overpack, but that's okay. Remember, all this will take up space in your little hospital room, so try to

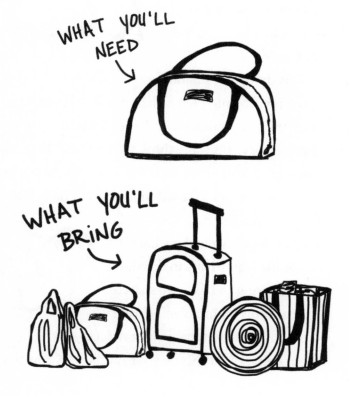

WHAT YOU'LL NEED

WHAT YOU'LL BRING

cut it back if you can. Here's my must-have list:

+ ID and insurance card for checking in, along
with some money

Your husband may have to pay for his own food, but yours will be included in your hospital stay.

+ Liquid food for energy

In case they only let you consume liquids during labor—honey straws, powder meal replacement shakes, etc.

+ A good camera

If your phone has an excellent camera, that works too. Just make sure you have enough storage and battery charge to take lots of pictures and videos. These pictures and videos are absolutely beautiful to revisit days and years later. (The videos we took on the way to the hospital and after the baby was born still make me cry.) You can even ask a tech or nurse to take pictures for you the actual moment the baby hits your chest. We are so grateful one of our nurses grabbed our camera and started clicking away without us even asking or realizing it at the time. Now we have a treasure trove of priceless photos of our faces in those first moments. (Just remember, you will be naked. Needless to say, these won't all be frame-worthy.)

+ Cell phone charger
+ One or two outfits for baby

Just onesies or sleepers—don't mess around with pants or sweaters yet, as baby will be swaddled all the time at this stage.

+ Toiletries

Shampoo, conditioner, body wash, body lotion, toothbrush, toothpaste, hair brush, hair ties, glasses, contact case and solution. Get ready for the best (and most-needed) shower of your life!

+ Two or three comfortable outfits

My go-to outfits were maternity leggings and shirts that would fit while five months pregnant. A long, comfy dress might also be nice, if you have one. Your tummy will be significantly smaller already, but you will still look pregnant. Bring something you feel good in but not your best outfit. Between the peeing newborn and the postpartum pelvic floor, there is fair potential for wardrobe casualties.

+ Comfortable nursing bra

I recommend no underwire. (For most breast-feeding at this point, you'll probably just have your bra and shirt completely off. It's hard to mess with that stuff until you get the hang of it).

+ Robe

If you're a robe lover, a robe can be a nice comfort. Just remember that it might get soiled, so I recommend a dark color and not your favorite one. I never brought one, as I felt more comfortable in stretchy maternity leggings and a loose top. Also, if you had a vaginal delivery, consider that your pelvic floor will require a ginormous pad at all times—maybe even with an ice pack in it! I always felt more comfortable with pants to make everything feel a little more secure and contained. However, I have enough friends who found their postpartum happy place in a robe, so I think it's worth adding to the list. It's personal preference.

+ One or two things to occupy yourself during down time

Consider a deck of cards or a book to read.

+ This book

Your letter for Month Nine is written specifically

for you to read during a quiet moment while you're still in the hospital. To save space in your bag, I've included a mini-journal after Month Nine for your convenience. The best time to capture your thoughts is while they are fresh in your mind, as you watch your new baby sleep.

+   Car seat installed in the car

The last thing you'll want to do the day you go home is futz around with a car seat for the first time. (Let's be honest, if you wait until that point, it will probably be your husband's job. Let's set him up for success and get it done ahead of time.) A nurse will likely teach you how to strap the baby in properly, so don't fret about that.

+   Blanket and car seat cover

Just in case the weather is cold or rainy, you'll want a way to protect that brand new baby from the harsh elements between the hospital door and your car door. If you know the weather will be hot, a thin blanket will be plenty. If it's winter in Wisconsin, you'll want a heavier blanket and maybe even a car seat cover to protect baby from wind. Don't worry, the nurses will be happy to advise you on how to dress your baby for whatever weather you're about to enter. This is one of those things I felt really clueless about, as do many new mamas.

The hospital will supply everything you need for nursing, as well as diapers, swaddle blankets, baby hats, and pelvic floor or incisional care, so don't bother packing any of that. They'll probably even let you take home the swaddle blankets and leftover diapers, pads, disposable underwear, numbing spray, etc. I would have a bag of large and extra-large pads ready at home beforehand though, as a vaginal delivery means bleeding will continue for three to six weeks. Yeah. I know. But the baby is really cute!

BRINGING IT HOME (THE LETTER, NOT THE BABY!)

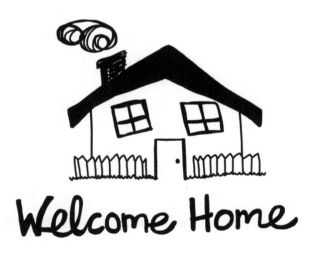

LETTERS TO THE EXPECTING MAMA

Whew! That was a lot of heavy information. Know that you can do this, dear friend! Remember that the pain we suffer during childbirth is the direct result of sin. (Genesis 3:16) It's something every childbearing woman since Eve has had to endure. You are not alone! Please reach out to a trusted friend if you need reassurance.

More importantly, remember that the curse connected with childbirth was also accompanied by the promise of a Savior. (Genesis 3:15) Remember that the suffering we deserve (at an eternal level) was placed on Jesus. He had the power to overcome unfathomable pain and even death in our place. For you. For me. What better way to understand how much Jesus loves us than during the unparalleled endeavor of birthing a child! Think about it. While you battle pain and discomfort for the sake of your coming child, it doesn't begin to compare to the pain and suffering Christ took on for you. That love is incomprehensible.

If you were the only person on Earth who needed saving, He would still come to save you. That's how much He loves you, lady. He will surely help you overcome this earthly suffering and reward you in so many ways when it's over. Lean on His promises for strength and perseverance, and trust that He will deliver...pun intended!

You are going to be okay, and as always, His plan for your special day is for your good and the good of those surrounding you. Let that brilliant light of yours shine. No matter what happens, He's got you, girl. He's protecting you and that baby. He's so excited for you to feel that sweet precious miracle against your skin; to marvel at His amazing creation, designed completely and uniquely for you and your husband. He is so excited to show you what He's made for you!

Give God the wheel.

You've got this, mama tiger!

Love, Kristen

"There is a
river whose streams
make glad the city of God,
the holy place where the Most
High dwells. God is within her,
she will not fall; God will help
her at break of day."

—Psalm 46:4-5

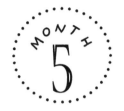

Relationship Maintenance

My dear friend,

YOU'RE ANOTHER MONTH CLOSER TO meeting your little one. You're over halfway there! You've seen your baby on the big screen ultrasound. Isn't it amazing how much you can see on that computer screen? You watched blood flowing through the heart and the umbilical cord and saw the size of the tiny organs. It's mind-blowing! You are so blessed to be pregnant in this day and

age when you have access to this kind of technology.

How breath-taking was it to actually *see* your child's heartbeat?

Did you cry? I'm crying!

God's designs are so beautiful.

You are so beautiful.

Do you ever make yourself smile? Seriously, do you ever catch a glimpse of yourself walking past a mirror, then back up to do a double take and think, "Dang, I look good!"? If you don't, you should. Because you do look good. You really do. Keep up the good work, mama!

This month, we're going to shift our focus away from baby and instead focus on the amazing new parents. I'm sure you've heard rumors of how a marital relationship can be rocked—in both good ways and bad—by having a baby. The rumors are true.

There's no denying that a marriage is affected by adding a new life to the mix—a third wheel, if you will. This is not just true for first-time parents. Every new life that joins a family will shift the dynamic and create some need for adjustment from all parties. In my experience, however, I found the first one to be the most dramatic.

Think about how you spend your day. How much time do you spend with your husband? How much time do you spend alone? There's a reason people say, "I can't remember life before the baby." Although, from my experience, I would say, "I can't remember what we did with our time before the baby."

Everything changes—how you wake up, when you wake up, how much sleep you get at one time, how much time you have alone with your husband, how much energy you have, where you can go, etc. All these things and more will be affected by that beautiful new life.

Let me assure you, it's totally worth it!

Life will stabilize again. There are a ton of wonderful, positive changes you'll experience because a child is now part of your life. As I mentioned in the previous letter, you and your husband will share a bond like never before because of the things you'll conquer together as parents.

It's going to be a shock to the system, but it's normal. If your struggles make you feel like you're on a deserted island without anyone to help you, know that you are not alone. Everybody goes through it.

My pastor once told me that the fifth year of marriage is typically the most difficult. Why? Because that's normally the time when babies start entering the picture. After my own seven years of marriage, I would agree with him on that.

So, this edition of Kristen's unsolicited advice is all about maintaining a great relationship with your husband, despite the speed bumps that lie in your path. For now, I'll stick to the pre-baby relationship stuff. I'll include post-baby stuff in the postpartum prep letter which is coming in a couple months. Get psyched!

RELATIONSHIP MAINTENANCE

My husband describes the length of time that a baby affects your lives together (in undesirable

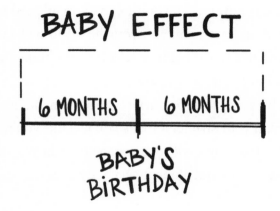

ways) as the six months before birthday and the six months after birthday. (I raise my brow at this estimation, but I guess he's the one who's had to deal with the hormonal shifts I may not have noticed at the time.) This is probably truer with subsequent pregnancies, unless your first one is particularly rough. With subsequent pregnancies, the effects of the pregnancy will be compounded by simultaneously caring for a toddler, so naturally you may feel more affected (and exhausted) the next time around.

Nevertheless, there are changes a man notices in his wife—and therefore in their relationship—during this timeframe, regardless of which child is on the way.

Sex

Let's face it, sex is not quite the same. There's a baby in the way. You may feel large and unattractive. You shouldn't, but sometimes you just do. You may be exhausted. Or, on the flip side, thanks to the hormones, you may feel extra excitable, in which case, good for you (and your husband)!

Consider the following thoughts to help keep that fire burning:

Never doubt your own beauty or your man's desire for you. He certainly doesn't. If you don't believe me, ask him.

There is something about the fact that your current predicament was caused by the two of you having sex that makes having sex again now all the more exhilarating. Ride that wave and have fun with it!

Find humor in the way being pregnant alters the things you are capable of during sex. It really is funny, isn't it? And irritating. But also funny. Kind of. Just laugh, dang it!

As always, prioritize this intimacy with your husband. Most likely, it's really important to him and his sense of normalcy, especially with the shockwave coming. It's a key way for both of you to maintain your closeness, your passion, and for lack of a better word, your youthfulness. Unfortunately, pregnancy and child rearing can make you feel… well, old. Sex is a great way to rekindle the romance that brought you together in the first place—and led you to make a baby.

Consider that everything about your nine months of pregnancy revolves around you and baby: your feelings, your discomforts, your symptoms, your doctor appointments, etc. And for good

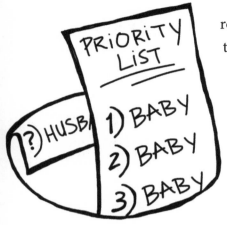

reason—you're going through a *lot* of things he'll never fully understand. At the same time, consider that this may lead your husband to feel like he's playing second-fiddle; like all his own feelings and desires are trumped by yours simply because you're the one who's pregnant. It goes a long way to show him you still want to be intimate with him. It tells him that his needs have not been forgotten, and that they are still important to you too. Respecting his needs and feelings, just as you want him to respect yours, is essential to the emotional health of your family unit. You need him, and he needs you.

Focusing some attention on him in this way will mean so much to him—and likely cause him to feel more compelled to return that love in ways that are important to you, like getting the baby's room ready on time. (See the coming section on nesting.) I hope this doesn't sound manipulative. Showing your love in any form should be sincere, not coercive. But it's true that sustained love is an action, not a feeling. The feelings result from the actions.

Savor opportunities to soak in all that closeness in this sweet space you have before baby arrives. It's just you and your man for a short while yet. As excited as you are to meet this baby, you still might look back from time to time and miss this dynamic duo when times were simpler.

Mood Swings

As much as we wish it weren't true, we have to admit that pregnancy can be like our own hormonal tilt-a-whirl, and it does make things harder for our faithful hubbies. This isn't to say we can help it. It's just part of the reality of pregnancy.

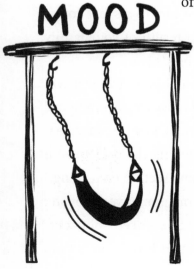

I remember one evening, long before I was pregnant myself, I was at a girls' night with a bunch of ladies who were slightly older than me. One lady, far along in her pregnancy, was giving us a hilarious rendition of the emotional overflow she had let loose on her husband a few days earlier. I could almost see her puddle of tears as she reenacted how she asked her husband through breathless sobs, "Why (sniff) do (sniff) you (sniff) still (sniff) love (sniff) meeeee?" We were laughing hysterically as she admitted to some of the ridiculous things pregnancy caused her to do.

As silly as the question was, she needed to hear the right answer in that moment to feel validated in her emotional struggle. Our husbands can be so good at this, but they can also be deer in the headlights at times.

Even if we can't fight the hormones, here are some tips for keeping your relationship intact in spite of them:

It's meaningful to our guys when we can own up to the inevitable and thank them for being such resilient shock absorbers.

Similarly, ask for forgiveness when you know you were hard to handle—short fused, poor reaction to an innocent comment, harsh, confusing, all-around difficult to keep up with emotionally, etc.

Remind him how much you need him. Tell him how much it means to you to feel supported when you're having trouble. Be direct. Let him know exactly what types of gestures uplift you. Hugs? Words of encouragement? Help with the dishes? He'll probably be much more successful if he knows what you're thinking, and if you, in return, let him know how much his support was appreciated.

It's okay, friend. Your husband loves you, for better and for worse. He knows pregnancy can be hard for you, as wonderful as it is. He knows your body is going through an awful lot. He won't hold hormones against you—even though he will definitely tease you about them at some point. Hopefully he waits until enough time has gone by that it won't be upsetting.

Nesting

I hated the word nesting. It made me feel like an animal. As if a pregnant woman doesn't feel like that already. So let's call it what it is: getting your home ready for another inhabitant. One who needs a *lot* more stuff than the current inhabitants. One who currently has no stuff at all. One whose future bedroom needs to be ready by an unknown delivery date and is currently full of dad's old military antique collection and gun arsenal. (At least the baby will be well-defended.) Honestly, was it that absurd to want the future nursery cleaned out before hunting season so I could fill it with all things baby (while I was still mobile, energetic, and home alone anyway) BEFORE the month the baby was due? (Insert frantic panting!)

Needless to say, I think nesting is a term made up by men to make us *think* 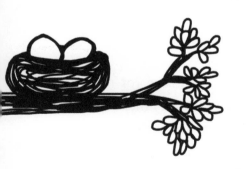 we're being hormonal and ridiculous about preparing the house, so that we'll stop asking them to help. I really don't think my requests were that outlandish. Eh, we'll never know for sure. It's still a sensitive topic in our house. Mainly because, regardless of who has the clearer memory of the situation, I don't enjoy feeling like an animal.

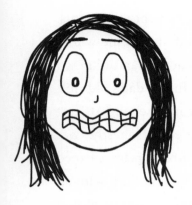

Anyway, I'm only listing this in the relationship maintenance letter because my husband claims nesting was one of the challenges to our relationship when I was pregnant. Getting your home ready for baby is important. Your stress level will be lowered knowing you have a special place for baby when it's time to come home. I'm not just talking about the nursery. It's normal to want your whole house to feel cozy and ready for a family of three. It's your maternal instinct kicking in, just the way God designed it!

If your husband is gently suggesting (or making fun of you, depending on his style) that you're going overboard, explain to him why this is all so important to you, but do also consider that you *might* be going overboard. Perhaps you're not, but do him the favor of at least considering.

Find peace in knowing that even if the nursery has the wrong color paint, or the baby comes before the rocking chair gets delivered, or even if the crib isn't put together in time, you already have everything you need for this baby—right now, today, as you read this. Love and Jesus. The rest will come!

love & Jesus

THE REST WILL COME

As a side note, baby-proofing the house really isn't necessary until the baby is 6-8 months old, when he or she can sit up, pull up, and crawl around and grab things. Feel free to do that if you're bored and need something to occupy yourself, but if you have a long to-do list, put baby-proofing at the bottom.

If you feel the need to scrub the kitchen floor on your hands and knees, just to know it's clean, go ahead and do it! No shame! Get it done, girl!

Let me offer one final suggestion regarding nesting (grrr, that word again!). It's a *really* great idea to make some freezer meals about two months before your due date. Make it a girls' day, have your mom or a couple friends over, and crank out a bunch of freezer meals. I recommend one to three batches of five different freezable recipes to get you through the first few weeks

MEAL #1 EAL #2

while you get your feet under you again. Cooking dinner is the *last* thing you are going to be thinking about those first couple weeks with a new baby. You'll be so glad you have meals ready to go in the freezer! My husband didn't knock my nesting when we were eating great meals three days after I gave birth. Just sayin'.

Communication

As always, communication is so important in keeping you and your spouse on the same page. Some guys are great at diving into discussions about their hopes, dreams, fears, and frustrations. Others might need some gentle coaxing. Don't get upset if your husband doesn't go nuts over the idea of having a conversation about how the near-perfect relationship with his beautiful bride will be challenged in the coming months.

Give him some time, and make sure you choose an appropriate time and place to discuss heartfelt things. Plant the seed, as my husband likes to say. Try not to sideswipe him with deep questions before he realizes this is on your mind. Instead, you could start by telling him some of your own feelings, and then express genuine interest in his. Make sure he

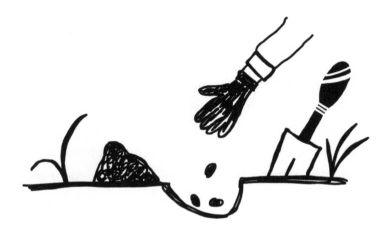

knows he's the most important person in your life. Let him know that you want this experience to bring you closer together, not drive you apart.

Here are a few questions that can help get a conversation going:

+ I'm worried about [fill in the blank]. Is there anything you're worried about?
+ Do you think we are doing a good job helping each other? Are we meeting each other's needs right now? If not, what can we do better?
+ What are your expectations for how our roles might change once baby comes (temporarily or long-term)?
+ How do you think our relationship might change after the baby comes?

+ What are some things you think we might struggle with most?

If you can speak openly about these fears, worries, and expectations in the months and days before baby arrives, you can keep those things fresh in your minds as you embark on the first weeks and months of parenting together. Hopefully you'll be able to understand one another's perspective better during those times than if you'd never talked about it. Additionally, pray about these things together. Ask God to calm your worries, help you both adapt to all the upcoming changes, and support each other through the challenges.

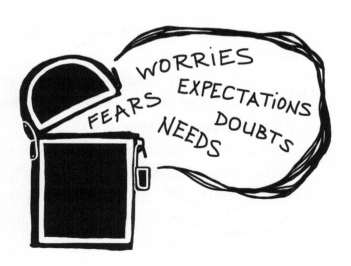

It might be helpful to share insight with him regarding the help you'll need once baby gets here. I remember being shocked at how little I could accomplish in a day besides simply responding to the newborn. Normal, daily tasks like washing dishes, making dinner, doing laundry, *showering...* they just won't get done, no matter how badly you want to keep up with them. You're going to need his help.

Phil has told me that this was one of the things he wasn't expecting. He knew I'd need more help than usual, but he had no idea how much! I'll never forget the love I felt for him the day we brought our first daughter home. He sent me to bed to nap while she was asleep. When I woke up to feed her, I saw that Phil had washed the dishes, cleaned the kitchen, and tidied up the living room despite being pretty tired himself. I was so thankful for that act of service—especially that he did it without me asking. (To be honest, I didn't even notice these things needed to be done!)

Likewise, he may be able to predict specific needs that he'll have during the coming months—things that maybe you've never considered. It's good for you to know these things now because it's easy to let the world revolve around baby to the point that you lose track of your best friend. Telling each other what you think you'll need (which may be different than before) will help you love each other to your highest potential during this time.

Sleep

We already know you can be short on quality sleep during pregnancy, whether it's due to discomfort, a busy brain, or the infuriating need to pee during the night. Keep in mind, your husband's sleep is probably being affected too. He might be waking up every time you roll over or get out of bed (because let's face it, you're not very graceful). He might have a lot on his mind, just like you do.

Remember that lack of quality sleep can make the waking hours harder, tempers hotter, and frustrations easier to surface. Be patient with each other, use your body pillow, refer to chapter three, and have some great sex.

Just for fun, here's my pro tip for improving gracefulness and efficiency of rolling over in bed: Move your *legs and pelvis* first, and your torso will follow. Happy abs!

As Always, You Got This!

Friend, you and your husband are going to be just fine. The fact that you just read this entire letter about relationship maintenance speaks to how much you care about it. As with all things in life, if your relationship is centered on Christ and His love, there will be nothing the three of you can't handle.

Pregnancy is a great time to cherish one another and make the most of every moment you have together, just the two of you. Enjoy dreaming of the future together, and revel in the excitement of knowing your baby is on the way!

When you got married, you knew the wedding day was the easiest part. You knew harder challenges would come—in the first year, the fifth year, the fortieth year—and you vowed before God to love each other anyway.

Having a baby is such a wild ride, but you share a coaster cart with your best friend! Remember that's what you are—the deepest form of best friends known to man. You are

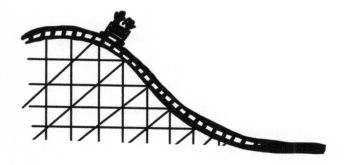

partners, lovers, and soul mates matched by God himself. You have each other's backs. You are armed with humility, forgiveness, and the love of a Savior who sets the most excellent example for you to follow. This baby will make you stronger and will teach you selflessness and love that you never knew before—for the baby and for each other.

As you get close to your due date, watch your wedding video or flip through the photos together one evening. Remember every moment that made you laugh, smile, and cry. Remember what it felt like to hold his hand when his touch still gave you butterflies. Hold fast to those memories as you

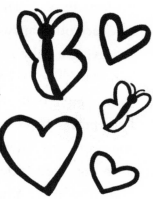

navigate this uncharted new season of life side by side. That's your man, and he always will be. You're in this together. You got this, guys!

Love, love, and more love!

Love, Kristen

"Be
completely
humble and gentle;
be patient, bearing with
one another in love. Make
every effort to keep the unity
of the Spirit through
the bond of peace."
—Ephesians 4:2-3

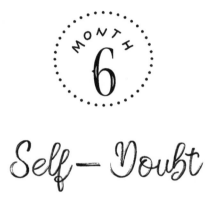

MONTH

6

Self – Doubt

My dear friend,

HAVE YOU HAD IT YET? THE MINOR PANIC attack in your favorite department store when you watched in disbelief as a mom totally lost control of her kids? Which reminded you of last week, when you heard that kid screaming in church and felt so bad for those parents. Which reminded you of that time in that place when you almost hit a kid with your car because he was running wild through the parking lot? And all at once you found yourself frozen in the kids clothing department, holding a

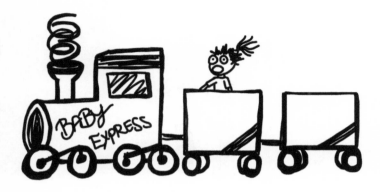

tiny newborn onesie, thinking, "Oh, God, I can't do this. Get me off this train. Put this kid back where it came from, or so help me! (Did images of Mike Wazowski of *Monsters, Inc.* just pop into your head? You're welcome.) I'm not ready. I thought I was, but I'm not. I have no idea what I would do in any of those situations. I need more time; I need to read so many parenting books; I need to talk to my pastor about his nine angelic children and document his entire parenting strategy; I need to commit at least a year of my life to solid prayer, and..."

Now I'm having a panic attack!

Take a deep breath, sister. Just...*breathe.*

SELF-DOUBT

I will never forget how my college biology professor described the experience of being pregnant. She stood in front of the lecture hall with a belly that expanded weekly. "It's like going up the first big hill on a rollercoaster," she said. "One second you're thinking, 'I'm so excited, I'm so excited!' and the next second you're thinking, 'I wanna get off! I wanna get off! I wanna get off!'"

So accurate, right?

Self-doubt is normal, and the fact that you have it means you care. Step one of being a good mom... *check*!

Furthermore, you should know this letter is by far the most difficult for me to write, simply because self-doubt doesn't go away. Do you know how hard it is to write advice on a topic you don't feel like you've mastered?

HOW TO OVERCOME SELF-DOUBT

HMM...

I don't believe self-doubt is a bad thing, as long as it's coupled with faith and trust in God. Without faith and trust, self-doubt can cripple you into becoming the dreaded helicopter mom or worse—the mom who gives up and checks out somewhere along the line.

Self-doubt will keep you humble. It will remind

you that, as hard as you strive to be the perfect woman, wife, or mom, you are still a flawed, sinful human being. Self-doubt will remind you that you'll never be completely self-sufficient. You need grace.

Pictures of friends' beloved babies on social media can make you feel as though motherhood will be a blissful state of smiles and giggles, and that you should be striving for this freeze-framed perfection. Ask any of those mamas how many failed attempts there were in the effort to capture those perfect moments. Every time I commend my pastor's wife on her amazing parenting, she smiles, but insists that she has plenty of failures that aren't seen in the church pews.

I believe it's healthy for children to see that their parents have weaknesses and sin. How can you tell them that everyone is sinful and needs Jesus' grace and forgiveness to get to heaven but then try to pretend you are not one of those people? How can a child take the importance of forgiveness seriously if they never see it demonstrated by their parents? It's easy to feel like they won't respect you if you admit your faults. In reality, they will see that you love them enough to be honest, even about your own faults. They will see words backed up by actions.

Here's the bottom line: it's okay to admit fault, and it's okay to be flawed. It's good to demonstrate the need for repentance and forgiveness and then model the appropriate response to grace. Namely, that you strive to do better out of thankfulness for that grace!

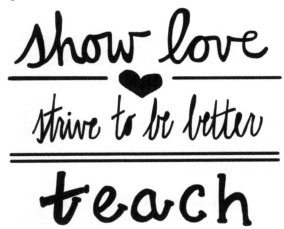

$$\frac{show\ love}{strive\ to\ be\ better} = teach$$

Flaws Turn Us to Christ

Children are God's way of giving parents a tiny glimpse of how frustrating His job can be.

I've had so many moments during these last three years of being a mom that made me pause and think, "This must be how God feels when I do X, Y, or Z—Hmm, I'm kind of a pain."

For example, when I tell my toddler for the

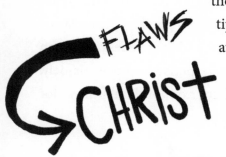

thousandth time not to tip her chair backward at the dinner table, yet she looks right at me and does it again, I think to myself, "If she just understood what would happen if I wasn't holding the front of the chair down, she would respect what I'm telling her!"

Which then leads me to think, "How many times has God held the chair for me while I kept doing something stupid?"

Here's another one: Like all moms, I give, give, *give* of myself every moment of every day to care for my children's every need. When I'm repeatedly met with a barrage of crying, whining, and defiance, I think, "Why are they treating me like this? Don't they see how much I do for them? Don't they understand how much I love them?"

I then realize this is how God must be feeling, multiplied by every person who ever lived.

Just as God's relationship with man suffered

dramatically after the fall into sin, so parenthood became a much harder job as well. Think of the Israelites as they wandered in the desert. Everything they needed literally fell from heaven, but still they whined to God that they wanted something else. Time and time again, God proved to them that He had things under control, only to watch His children run the other way. Once I became a mom, I finally got a true glimpse of how God must feel when his people act that way.

As always, though, God doesn't stop with law and the gloom and doom of sin. Children are also His way of showing us the beauty of grace.

I have never met a grown person as capable of forgiveness as my toddler. I wish I could say I never screw up as a mom, but the truth is that becoming a mom has revealed my flaws like nothing I've ever experienced.

In the heat of a power struggle with a toddler, I've made wrong decisions. In the exhausted haze that follows restless nights, I've made wrong decisions. In the moments when my children test me to see how I will react, I've made wrong decisions.

There are times when I'm convinced my wrong decisions will leave emotional scars that my children will never outgrow. Sometimes I'm afraid

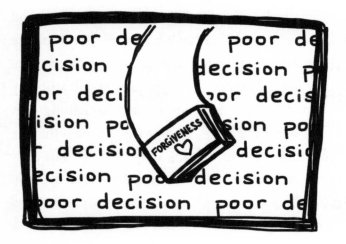

there is no way my child will continue to love me like she did before.

But they do. Within mere seconds. They always do.

My daughters, in their sweet youth, reflect the grace of God as plainly as I have ever seen it. The ease with which my children can shift from incessant, hurting tears to pure, genuine forgiveness brings me to my knees.

How am I worthy of such boundless love?

I've been overcome with tears more than once as I'm wrapped in my toddler's arms, lost in wonder at the sheer power of grace in such a simple form. It leads me back to Christ every time. It reminds me that He continues to shower me with grace despite my recent lack of prayers, my selfish heart, and my impatience and mismanagement of these precious lambs He has given me. In the next moment, my toddler is leading me off to play Legos like nothing happened.

Can you imagine the freedom your heart would feel if you could forgive so quickly? The things God can teach us through our children are remarkable, if we pause long enough to listen.

Okay, now that I've emptied another tissue box…

Let's break down some components of self-doubt and learn how to conquer them!

SELF-DOUBT #1: I'M NOT READY.

One of my favorite cliché questions to a pregnant woman is, "So, are you ready?"

There is absolutely no way anyone can ever be ready for their first baby. Ready is what you are when you are fed, clothed, and on your way out the door for work. Ready is what you feel when you've gone through your pre-game routine and are standing at center court, poised for tip-off.

Ready is not what you feel when you go into

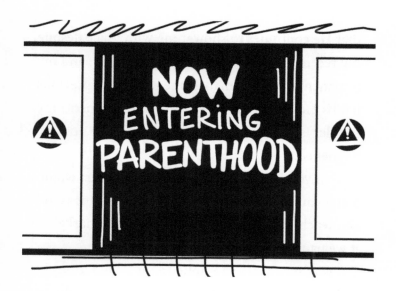

the hospital one day responsible for one life and come out a couple days later responsible for two. No matter how many books you've read ahead of time, you can't possibly anticipate exactly what it will be like to hold that long-awaited child—*your* child—in your arms, knowing that the simple presence of that tiny creature is about to flip your world upside down. Don't worry, no one expects you to feel ready for that!

You can find comfort in knowing that the One who has been sculpting that child from the moment of conception will not suddenly abandon him or her at birth. He continues to love and protect that child, even in ways that you can't. As a human being, you have lots of limitations. You are powerless in so many circumstances of earthly life. Having a child reveals your human shortcomings like nothing else. It's an incredibly powerful time for God to show you how much you need Him, and all the ways He can strengthen and provide for you.

You may not feel ready, but God is ready to take your hand and guide you through this!

It's interesting to me how God cleverly structured a child's development in a way that allows the new mama to keep up. At first, a baby cannot do anything but lie in one place. God knew that a brand new mom has enough on her plate with her own healing, and that energy and sleep are low during this phase. Therefore, a newborn baby is immobile. You're welcome. Love, God.

Once you get the hang of life again, baby starts to roll—a friendly warning that you will no longer be able to set baby down and trust that the little rascal will still be there when you turn around. You'll have to start planning ahead a bit more. Next, baby will sit up and crawl,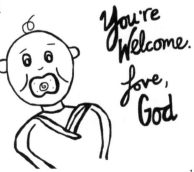

followed by pulling up to stand, and finally walking and running.

Each new phase requires an added level of alertness and forward thinking from mom. But the fact that God gives you some time to adapt to each one prepares you for what's coming next. In that respect, you don't have to be ready for everything right away.

SELF-DOUBT #2:
I DON'T KNOW WHAT I'M DOING.

When you start feeling clueless, take heart knowing that you are not alone!

Every seasoned mama started out as a relatively ignorant young woman who had never changed a diaper before—even Eve, the mother of all the living. She had the ultimate journey of naïve motherhood. Can you imagine if you were the first one who had to figure out what labor contractions were? The first one to wonder how in the world that baby was going to exit her body? The first one to figure out how to get a screaming, hungry baby to latch properly? The first one to figure out how to fasten an absorbent leaf around a baby's butt? The first one to navigate every new stage of development and try

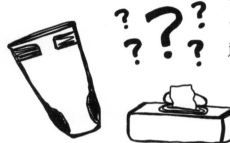

to figure out whether it's worthy of concern or just normal behavior?

Sure, maybe Eve had a superhuman trust in God. After all, she had spoken with Him directly at one point. Still, since she was the one who had experienced the fall into sin firsthand, I have a feeling her doubts and worries were as human as the rest of ours. Can you imagine how much she might have enjoyed having a girlfriend to commiserate with? I mean, I know she and Adam were close, but I'm sure it just wasn't the same.

You are so blessed to have all sorts of resources to help you navigate the world of parenthood. You have countless books, online articles, forums, mommy groups, friends, family, your own mama, and the Bible to guide you through this crazy time in life. Even your doctor is only a phone call or an email away. If there was ever a time to be pregnant, this is the jackpot. Don't be

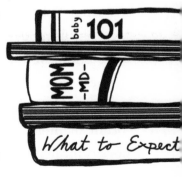

afraid to use these resources and have confidence that you aren't alone in your journey!

Of course, there will be times when you'll find yourself a little too dependent on online resources. If you find yourself convinced that your child's fever of 100.5 is a rare and deadly bacteria picked up from that grain of sand he put into his mouth two weeks ago, remember that sometimes the ease with which you can access information on the internet is not always the best thing. Trust God and your pediatrician instead.

Even with the wisdom of those who have gone before, motherhood is still going to have unique challenges because no two children are exactly the same. Ask my pastor's wife, the one with nine kids. She'll smile sweetly and tell you that as soon as you think you have motherhood all figured out, the next child will come and your tactics will have to totally change. Likewise, just because a whole forum of moms adamantly suggest one strategy doesn't mean it's guaranteed to work for your child (but it might be worth a try).

I don't mean for this to sound scary. I mean for it to be a reassurance that it's totally normal to feel like you don't know what you're doing.

Motherhood is the epitome of flying by the seat of your pants and learning as you go. It's a series of constant experiments, testing to see what works and what doesn't, making subsequent adjustments, big and small.

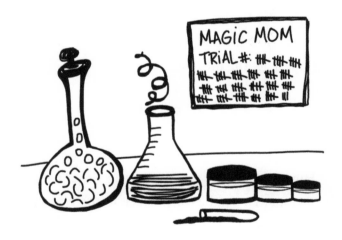

Most importantly, don't forget your *best* resource—your own Heavenly Father. In all things, pray. If you don't even know what you should be praying for, just fold your hands and groan. Seriously, it's in the Bible!

"The Spirit helps us in our weakness. We do not know what we ought to pray for, but the Spirit himself intercedes for us through wordless groans. And he who searches our hearts knows the mind of the Spirit, because the Spirit intercedes for God's people in accordance with the will of God. And we know that in all things God works for the good of those who love him, who have been called according to his purpose." —Romans 8:26-28

There you have it. When in doubt, just groan, girl! He'll get the message.

SELF-DOUBT #3: I'M NOT GOOD ENOUGH.

How many times have you seen negative adult behaviors that can be traced back to the way a person was raised?

That girl didn't have enough love from her dad.

That guy spent way too much time in front of a screen instead of at the dinner table.

That girl could never live up to the ridiculous expectations of her mother.

That guy was never taught to respect women.

That girl is so entitled. Her parents never told her no.

In a world full of sin, there's no denying that raising a child is challenging. There's no denying there are ways that you and I as parents *can* do our children long-term harm. It's truly terrifying! One of my worst fears of motherhood is that there will be some type of irreversible fault that my kids develop as a result of how I'm raising them, which will negatively impact the rest of their lives. What a horrible fear!

This is Satan whispering, "You're not good enough."

Do not listen to this voice. Like everything Satan says, it's a lie.

Instead, listen to the still, comforting voice of Jesus, the calm in the storm that is the world around us.

> "Have I not commanded you? Be strong and courageous. Do not be afraid; do not be discouraged, for the LORD your God will be with you wherever you go." —Joshua 1:9-10

> "Take my yoke upon you and learn from me, for I am gentle and humble in heart, and you will find rest for your souls. For my yoke is

easy and my burden is light." —Matthew
11:28-30

You prayed for this child, and God answered. (If
you didn't pray to have a child right now, God knew
this was the perfect time to give you one anyway.)
He does not say "yes" to requests that He knows are
not good for those who love Him (Romans 8:28).
He said "yes," dear friend. You are good enough. He
clearly thinks so.

Practically speaking, then, how can you actually
be good enough? It's really not as complicated as it's
made out to be.

It's just love!

It doesn't come
about by just saying
you love your kids. It
happens when you
demonstrate that love
by putting their needs
above all else. (This is not
to be confused with always
giving them whatever they
want).

The adults in the examples
above are probably people who

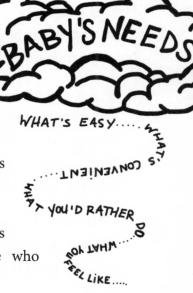

didn't have present and attentive moms and dads, who did their best to model Christ's love day in and day out. Parenting is really hard work, but when it comes down to it, it's just genuine love.

This might mean applying loving discipline when a child behaves inappropriately.

This might mean making a child wait for something he wants.

This might mean enforcing a consequence for defiant behavior, even when you know the child will scream and cry.

This might mean offering a choice between a healthy snack or no snack at all, despite incessant whining for more cookies.

This might mean choosing the more difficult route in the moment, knowing the long-term benefits.

This might mean using that last ounce of energy to read to or play with your children rather than plopping them in front of a screen again.

As an aside, plopping your kids in front of the TV once in a while for needed time or sanity for yourself does *not* make you a bad mom. The key is to reserve it for when it's really needed, especially when the kids are super young. There will be times when you have to, say, pack for a big move, and it's literally impossible without some kid-friendly distraction from the tube. It's okay, mama. Their brains won't melt! They'll probably even learn something if you pick the right show. My older

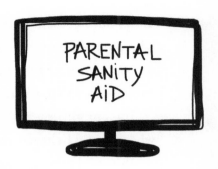

daughter's ability to verbalize colors suddenly improved after we let her watch *Little Baby Bum* on Netflix for the first time. Be forewarned, it's crazy how addictive screens can be and how content kids are to sit there like zombies and watch them. In our house, we really have to keep it as a special treat, or that's all the girls ever want to do. Be careful with this very slippery slope.

Love also means all the fun things! Hugs and kisses. Saying "I love you." Saying "I'm proud of you." Special experiences and treats. Reading books together. Rocking and singing songs about Jesus at bedtime. Belly laughs. Teaching about Jesus' love. These are the things your child will remember about growing up in your home, and about having you for a mama.

A childhood filled with love, soaked in and poured out, is all your sweet baby needs to become the young man or woman you hope and pray for. You provide that with God's help because you're...well, YOU!

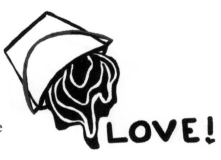

LOVE!

SELF-DOUBT #4:
I DON'T THINK I CAN BALANCE WORK AND MOTHERHOOD AND STILL FEEL GOOD ABOUT BOTH.

Ugh. Such a real dilemma! It's been said that we are expected to work as if we don't have kids, and raise kids as if we don't work. This is a real struggle for so many mamas everywhere.

The key is not only to find the right fit in terms of days and hours of work, but also the right fit in the actual job itself.

I was very career-driven before having kids. The moment I got pregnant, I knew my priorities had shifted away from work and toward being home with my kids. I have a friend who was just the opposite. She got married with the full intention of being a stay-at-home mom. But once she had children, she felt drawn to pursue a career, so her

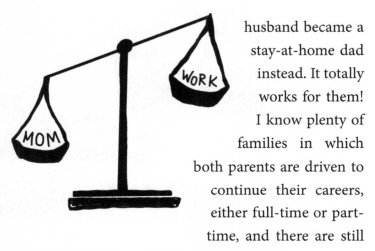

husband became a stay-at-home dad instead. It totally works for them! I know plenty of families in which both parents are driven to continue their careers, either full-time or part-time, and there are still several options for safe, quality childcare.

Everyone's situation is different. There are pros and cons to every decision you can make. So how will you know what your mom-work balance should look like?

Here are some good questions to ask yourself and discuss with your husband as you try to make these decisions:

Is continuing to work important to you?

How much fulfillment do you feel from what you do outside the home? How strongly do you feel about staying home more often and why?

What kind of lifestyle do you want for your family, and what will you need to do to achieve that?

If you know you want to stay home with your kiddos, would you be willing to sacrifice some other things about your lifestyle to make it happen?

If you really want to stay home with your child but also want to provide experiences that are costly—say, international travel—are you willing to work part-time for that if you have to? Would you rather tweak your budget in other ways so you don't have to work at all but still be able to keep travel options open?

Is the lifestyle you want or the things you're used to spending money on worth the extra time away from your kids? Once you have kids, maintaining the ability to afford these types of things might have to come at the cost of working more hours and spending less time with the kids. I'm thinking of things like the latest and greatest technological gadgets or the most luxurious vehicles, for example. I don't believe it's a bad thing to indulge in the blessings God has put on our earth. However, I do think it's worth taking a step back to analyze priorities.

What are your childcare options? Are you comfortable with those options?

Consider pros and cons of each option. Our kids are super close with their grandparents and my sister because of the one day per week they spend with each of them while I'm at work. However, as the babies grew to toddlers, we could tell they might benefit from a bit more interaction with other kids their age. We made sure to have some playdates with friends and started the kids in our church's daycare once a week, just to make sure they were getting some beneficial social time with their peers.

If you don't have family close enough to babysit but don't feel comfortable with the local daycare options, you could consider hiring a nanny. One of Phil's cousins nanny-shares with another family. The two families split the cost of the nanny, who comes to one of their homes each day. Their son gets social interaction with the other family's child every day, and the nanny is dedicated

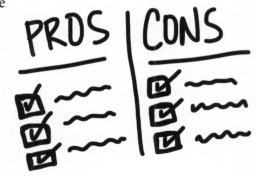

to helping the children meet milestones and all that good stuff. Cool!

How do you feel you can maintain your own identity?

Whoa, this just got deep! This is a question that is hard to answer before you've been a mama for a little while, and your answer may change depending what phase of motherhood you are in.

When I had my first daughter, I definitely wanted to be a stay-at-home mom. At the same time, I felt it was important to maintain my physical therapy skills. After all, it took a lot of hard work and education to achieve that, and helping others gave me a great sense of fulfillment. I chose to work two or three days a week, which was perfect, but I was always a little tempted to try staying home full time.

It wasn't until I had to be home full time for a few months during the COVID-19 lay-offs of 2020 that I real- ized I needed that outside piece of my identity. I give stay-at-home moms the greatest applause. I found that staying home with my kids 24/7/365 was more work than actually going to work. The ceaseless, day-to-day giving of myself got to me after a while. Phil still makes fun of me for the four-day stretch when I didn't shower. (No new baby to blame for that one.) There was a point during those few months when I actually looked forward to the one day a week that I helped my husband's crew install fences. Picture me carrying and pouring 60-pound bags of dry concrete, shoveling dirt for hours, digging up rocks with a post-hole digger, and becoming the first doofus employee to fall into a three-foot hole. That's what I looked forward to, just so I could step away from the perpetual role of caregiver for a day and have some unique time with my husband. I also looked forward to running errands when I could listen to podcasts without being interrupted. With the kids

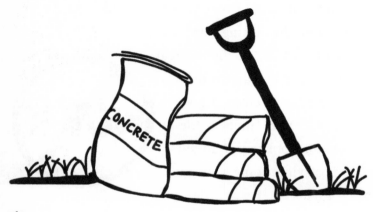

strapped in their car seats, I could briefly immerse myself in something for *me*.

This is when I realized that although being a mom was a huge and treasured part of my identity, there were pieces missing that I wanted to take back. I started making time for my hobbies of reading and writing, and eventually I got called back in to work my regular two days per week in the PT clinic. After adding these things to my plate, I actually felt more happiness and energy during my time at home with the kids. Being things besides a mom helped restore my sense of fulfillment and renewed the multi-faceted identity I believe God designed me to have.

I know many stay-at-home moms who are much hardier than me, who can embrace that challenging role with greater patience and perseverance than I can! However, I've found that even if they don't work outside the home, most moms do end up regaining some form of work or hobby that allows them to fulfill that need to have their own identities apart from being mamas. An Etsy or Instagram store, a blog, a mom/kid play group, a Bible study group, a town volleyball league, etc.

Whatever maintaining your own identity looks like for you (and it may change over time), remember that it's healthy to do something for *you* in addition to loving and caring for those precious babes. It's completely normal to feel that need. In no way does it mean that you don't love and cherish your kids to the max!

If you choose to work outside the home, will your type of work complement your time at home, or will it exacerbate your stress at home?

As soon as I had my first daughter, I knew my job at that time was no longer a good fit for me. I had worked in a clinic where I was expected to see two or three patients at a time, every hour, all day long. It was exhausting. Once I had a little one to chase around at home, I knew I did not want a job where I had to chase around patients as well, trying desperately to stay one step ahead of everyone. I found a new job working for a local hospital system in which I would be guaranteed to treat only one patient at a time. It was a much slower pace than my previous job, and it's exactly what I needed in a workplace at that point in life. I could focus my energy at work on the part that really fulfills me— quality patient care—and come home to my kids without my head already spinning.

I highly recommend considering the above

question when deciding what you want or need work to look like, as it may or may not be different than what has worked for you in the past. You need to enjoy your time away from the house as much as you

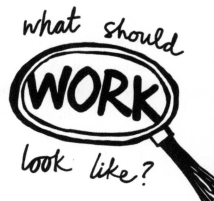

can, or it will deplete you pretty quickly. I pray you have the flexibility to be choosy and find something you really like to do!

These are some big questions that might be super frustrating if you don't know the answers yet. Try not to worry. If you feel like you've made the wrong decision, you can always change it.

You can look for a job that offers more flexibility or time off.

You can find a job where you can work from home.

You can quit your job altogether.

You can find a trustworthy daycare option and pick up more hours at work.

You can find a different job in the same field that better suits your current work needs.

There are a lot of options out there, so try not to

feel too stressed about finding the perfect fit right away. It's certainly ideal if you get it right the first time, but if not, it's going to be okay. You're not locking yourself in for life, and sometimes a refreshing change can be healthy too.

Keep in mind that the situation will likely change as the kids age. The kids will be in kindergarten by age five, and you'll have a lot more time on your hands. Of course, when they are in high school and if they're involved in extracurriculars, you may only have a few hours a day with them. (Pause here to shed tears or jump for joy, whichever comes naturally.) Finally, there will be empty nesting. (Tears! All the tears!) Do you want to leave some doors open for when you have more time to work? Do you think you may be able to pick up wherever you want when the time comes, even if you stop working completely in the meantime? All of these things will make a difference in your decision-making process.

Don't forget to pray. God will guide you to the right decisions at the right times.

SELF-DOUBT #5:
I WILL REALLY STRUGGLE
TO ADJUST TO THIS
COMING CHANGE.

Sudden change in your sleep patterns, sudden change in the relationship with your spouse, sudden change in available time, sudden change in so many parts of your life. It's normal to feel anxiety about how you'll deal with all of this change.

Take the unnecessary pressure off yourself right off the bat by admitting that you *are* going to struggle. Somehow, some way, these changes are going to be hard for you. Don't try to handle everything perfectly. It's impossible, and if that's your expectation going into this, you will feel like a failure. This thought makes me sad. Don't do it. You're not a failure!

I think what really matters here is how you *respond* to the struggle.

Lots of amazing things in this world exist as a direct result of immense struggle. When super-hot lightning strikes the right kind of sand, a glass tunnel is formed in the sand. Extreme combinations of heat and pressure within the earth yield the crystalized carbon atoms we know as diamonds.

My vegetable garden took off like magic after a massive summer storm (which is almost as cool as the formation of glass and diamonds). In the world of physical therapy, micro-traumas to muscle (a.k.a. weight training) slowly rebuild to create stronger, healthier muscle over time.

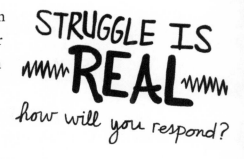

Dealing with all the coming changes at once seems mighty daunting. With God's fortitude and guidance, you *will* adjust and emerge stronger on the other side. You just will!

I wish I could offer deeper wisdom, but when I think back on how I did it, I don't even have an answer besides "I just did." These days, if both kids wake up once during the same night, I feel like a train hit me the next morning, and I wonder how in the world I ever survived getting up every two hours through the night to feed a newborn. You just pray, and nap, and God gets you through one day at a time until suddenly you don't remember what it was like to be up in the middle of the night. That will be a great day!

Here is my best advice for responding positively to the struggles:

+ Trust God and his promises to sustain you.

+ Accept help from friends and family, and don't be afraid to ask for it.

+ Acknowledge imperfections, but don't allow them to define your worth.

+ Communicate with your husband. Love your husband. Teamwork makes the dream work. When you struggle, reach for understanding, patience, and acts of love. Be humble when you know you have failed at these things. Try again, and ask him for the same.

+ Notice the ways God is strengthening you through the struggles. Write them on Post-It notes and tape them to your mirror. Let them be frequent reminders of the truly amazing mama that you are!

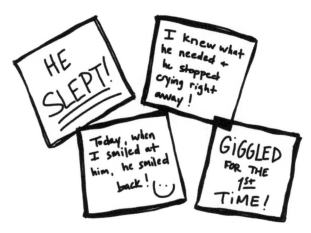

+ Talk to your network of other trusted mamas. Share your struggles with each other. Sometimes this allows a much-needed emotional release that leaves you feeling empowered and ready to take on another day!

+ Hold that precious babe in your arms and smell that sweet baby skin. Listen to *Safe and Sound* and *Unplanned* by Christian singer Matthew West. Grab the tissues, and get ready for a seriously renewed perspective. Never lose sight of the big picture—that amazing, miraculous gift that caused all this change. That little miracle will make every moment of struggle worthwhile!

God has placed your dear child into capable hands. He doesn't make mistakes!

Where your hands aren't capable, God's are.

With this knowledge, take a cleansing breath of fresh air, and smile. You are enough, and you're going to be the best mama ever.

Love you, my friend!

Love, Kristen

"May the God of hope fill
you with all joy and peace
as you trust in Him, so that
you may overflow with hope
by the power of the Holy
Spirit."

—Romans 15:13

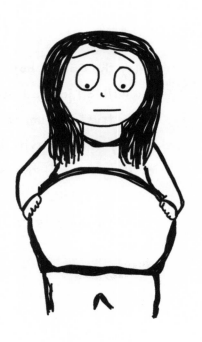

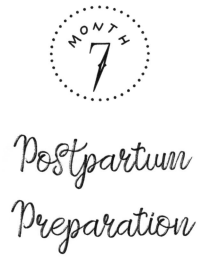

Postpartum Preparation

Dear friend,

YOU'RE IN YOUR THIRD TRIMESTER, mama! You are no doubt feeling the physical effects of being beautifully, unmistakably, "when's that lady going to pop" pregnant. You are no doubt reveling in the sage wisdom and advice of so many well-meaning folks. I'm guessing you're starting to face the reality of that special date that's creeping ever closer. The months on your calendar between now and your due date are down to two!

As you feel that date sneaking closer—wait, let's be real, it's not sneaking. You are hyper aware of exactly what day of pregnancy you are at and how many you have to go. There's nothing sneaky about baby #1.

Baby #2 will be the sneaky one.

Anyway, as the due date gets closer, you may find yourself thinking more and more about what it's going to be like in the weeks following the great birthday. When baby actually comes, how can you feel as prepared as possible to suddenly be a mom?

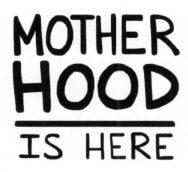

MOTHER HOOD
IS HERE

As I shared in my last letter, it's impossible to be completely ready for it. Nonetheless, having some pearls of wisdom (or commiseration) from a fellow mama can help. As I found out after that original note from my friend Anne, it made a huge difference in my postpartum experience to know I wasn't sailing through uncharted waters alone.

I want you to look back on this chapter the week you have your baby. Be reassured and encouraged by it if you start feeling overwhelmed.

Okay, buckle up—here we go!

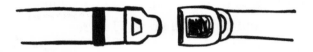

UNSOLICITED ADVICE FOR THE POSTPARTUM MAMA

Caring for a Newborn

Although you will be so in love with your newborn miracle, that doesn't mean he or she won't feel like a stranger to you in a lot of ways.

I felt like something was wrong with me because the bond with my firstborn didn't feel quite like I expected it to right off the bat. Love was there of course—but the intense, unconditional, deep bond that I expected actually took a few weeks to develop as I got to know her. None of my friends' Facebook birth announcements had ever mentioned this. I finally came to realize this can be normal after talking to one of my friends a year later. She described having the same feelings after the birth of her first child. It's hard to put into words, and maybe you will be one of those moms who will feel 110% bonded to baby from the start. Even if it doesn't feel as strong as you expect it to at first, that love and bond *will* grow! Have no doubt about that.

Another thing that surprised me after having my first child was how harsh it felt to be cried at. Newborn babies can be very dramatic. It's so easy to take it personally when you're trying your best to help your baby and all you get in return is screaming. Don't take it personally! That little newborn loves you more than anyone else in this world but doesn't know how to tell you yet.

If you need a second to step away and breathe, that's sometimes the best move even if baby has to cry in the crib for that moment. Babies can feel your stress, so sometimes it's good for you to take some time and space to feel God's restoring hand before you try tackling this challenge again. You and baby will both be better off for it in the end.

If you could use reassurance, talk to other moms. Be honest about your feelings and struggles. It's tempting to put on a brave face, but you'll find the most encouraging and revitalizing support comes from honest, vulnerable conversation. You are not alone!

Don't underestimate the power of physical support either. Accept help, always! If people offer meals, take them gladly! If family members offer to do something for you when they come visit the new baby, politely accept.

People who offer help are doing so because they get it. They know how incredibly hard it is to get anything done during this time, and they *want* to be a blessing to you and take a little off your plate. Let them tidy up your dinner dishes; let them fold your laundry as you chat with them; let them hold the baby while you take a nap. I have a friend who was bold enough to answer visit requests with, "Sure, if you help me do X, Y, or Z!"

It might be hard to imagine being that bold right now, but trust me when I say your capacity to do it all yourself will be nil for a while. Expect to have short to-do lists. I mean *really* short, like two or three simple things per day, such as "take a shower" and "do one load of essential laundry—i.e. burp cloths and bra liners."

It's easy to take it as personal failure when you feel like you live day after day without accomplishing anything substantial besides keeping your baby alive. This is not failure. This is success! It's literally your only job for the first few weeks after baby arrives while you figure things out and try to catch as much sleep as you can. That's it.

On that same note, it's worth mentioning that if you constantly try to do too much in the first couple weeks, you can actually be working your body too hard for it to heal.

After my second child was born, I thought, "This is round two. I know what I'm doing, and I have to do a better job of getting back to normal life right away this time around." Within the first week, I started running a fever and getting body aches and chills. I thought I was getting the flu, but sure enough, things went back to normal after a single day of resting and forgetting about keeping up with housework. I was just doing too much activity while my body was trying to heal and make breastmilk for my new baby. Take it slow, and take care of yourself.

It would sure help to be able to get more sleep, but you already know that's not going to happen with a newborn. You'll have to be up every two to three hours through the night to feed your newborn. You may need to keep baby upright for an additional 20-30 minutes after each feeding to prevent spitting up. This means you might be spending a lot of time fighting to stay awake in the dark as you rock your sleeping baby on your shoulder, while you're on the verge of falling asleep yourself. Since it's dangerous to fall asleep with a newborn, this can be quite a dilemma.

A trick that I recommend is to always have at least three things within arm's reach of the rocking chair: some snacks (breastfeeding makes you really hungry in the middle of the night), a water bottle (hydrate!), and your phone. Put the phone on the dimmest light setting, and use it to keep yourself awake. You can make lists of things you don't want to forget to do, watch quiet YouTube videos, research something you've been wondering about, respond to text messages, check up on your friends on Facebook, research vacation ideas—heck, start looking up ideas for the baby's first birthday party if you want to! Use it to engage your brain just enough to keep yourself awake and keep baby safe in your arms.

Eventually, you'll feel comfortable enough in your new-mama flow to start venturing out of the house with your newborn. Always plan a 15-30 minute buffer between the time you tell yourself you're going to leave the house with baby and the actual time you need to leave.

For example, if pre-baby Phil and Kristen left the house for church at 8:30 to get there for the 9:00 service, then post-baby Phil and Kristen will need to start loading up the car at 8:00 or 8:15. Why?

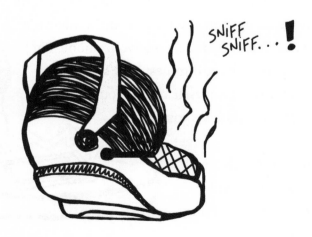

Because this is what will inevitably happen: Kristen is doing the 8:00-right-before-we-leave diaper change. Baby Behl pees on her, so Kristen has to change her clothes and clean pee off the floor and wall. Then, as Phil is loading Baby Behl in the car seat, he notices the unmistakable aroma of newborn poop, followed by visual confirmation up the back of the onesie. Craaaaaaaaap! (Pun intended.) Kristen rushes Baby Behl to the bathtub for a speed cleaning and outfit change number three. Finally, the whole family is clean, in the car, and pulling out of the driveway at 8:25. This is perfect, because it gives them a few extra minutes once they get to the church parking lot to gather the car seat and diaper bag from the backseat and get baby settled in the pew by the time church begins. Phew!

Honestly, you'll never have as much trouble getting out the door on time as you will with a newborn. Even while my kids are three and one-and-a-half, I still start loading everyone up 15 minutes before we actually need to leave, because it almost always takes longer than expected for one reason or another. And if you ask my husband, I'm still almost always running late.

Here's one last word to the wise for carting around a newborn: Always pack an extra change of clothes or two for the baby, expecting the first outfit will get soiled before you get back home. It's also not a bad idea to keep an extra change of clothes for *you* in the car. Assume that at some point you will get spit up on, peed on, or pooped on in public, and you'll be mighty thankful you have back-ups.

You will get the hang of having a child. I promise!

Breastfeeding

Breastfeeding is a journey that can be frustrating for you *and* baby and can really test your patience. It seems like it should be a natural thing, but there are a lot of intricacies to it. You and baby are both learning together. Be patient with each other as it's rare for both mama and baby to be really good at it the first time. Once you get the hang of it, if that's God's plan for you, it's an indescribable bonding experience between you and baby. It's something unique that only you, mama, can provide.

Breastfeeding is a beautiful thing, but it can be

horribly awkward in ways most people don't see. In the trial and error
of learning to do it right, your
boobs and nipples can really
struggle for a while. I'll share
insight from my experiences
to give you a good laugh and a
heads up.

ANOTHER
NEW
BESTIE

NIPPLE
CREAM

Your body doesn't start producing milk until a few days after
baby is born. I did not realize this. In
fact, it took a few days longer than it should have
for me before I realized what was going on. At first,
you'll just produce small quantities of a super nutritious substance called colostrum, which gets baby
through the first few days before milk is produced.

If baby's latch technique isn't spot on, you may
start to notice your nipples getting sore. Really sore.
Like, cringing when baby tries to latch because
you're being furiously pinched in the nipple for
the twentieth time that day. You only have about
an hour or two for your sorry little nipples to heal
before they have to undergo the horror again. Hey,
the kid has to eat! It's critical to get your newborn to
latch correctly in order to save yourself from miserable suffering.

When the real stuff does finally come in, your boobs will be gigantic and hard as rocks. What? Yes. Rocks. Somehow, I did not know this engorgement was coming. (Ick, there's another word that 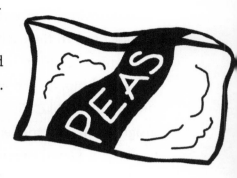 made me feel like an animal again.) I was completely caught off-guard and weirded out. Boobs that full felt *really* sore! I didn't have boob-shaped ice packs, so I walked around with bags of frozen peas in my bra for a couple days. I definitely felt attractive at that point. The things we do for our kids. Also, boob-shaped ice packs are a thing, and you should invest in a pair.

All this happens because your body doesn't know how much milk your baby is going to drink at first, so, to play it safe, it overproduces…a lot. If the discomfort is unbearable, you do have the option to use a pump to relieve some tension. You have to be careful if you do this, because your body doesn't recognize that it's being pumped for relief purposes and not because the baby is actually that hungry. This has potential to cause your body to keep producing excessive volumes of milk and prolong the engorgement phase. Typically, if you pump out just enough to take the edge off, you won't have any problems. Your body will figure it out within a week or two, and although you will still get really full when baby goes longer than usual without eating, it won't be as bad as engorgement.

Be patient if your baby is having trouble latching during this phase. Talk about being set up to fail—it's like trying to bite a basketball! Sometimes it even helps to hand-express (massaging your boob

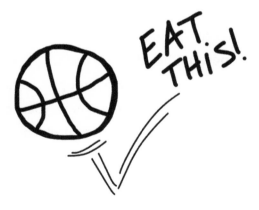

until milk comes out) beforehand to help baby latch better. It's like deflating that basketball.

Seriously, breastfeeding is so much weirder than most people realize! All at once, you'll be saying these things out loud like they're no big deal.

As an aside, I wouldn't be a good friend if I didn't

warn you: Breastfeeding boobs can start leaking at any time. Stepping out of a warm shower, having sex with your husband, etc. Be prepared! It's not uncommon to have a spontaneous letdown of milk if your baby goes longer than usual without eating, or if you experience a trigger that makes your body think it's feeding time. That's why those washable absorbent bra liners are super helpful.

If you are having trouble getting the hang of breastfeeding, lactation consultants can give you lots of tools and tricks for making the journey easier. They can teach you how to help your baby latch properly and how to hold the baby correctly for your postural health. They can supply you with nipple shields, nipple cream, and plastic cups that keep your shirt from rubbing against your sore nipples. Seriously, if you are having a problem with any aspect of breastfeeding, they can give you a solution. They can also help you understand and catch more serious issues like clogged ducts or mastitis. Don't be shy about getting professional help with this very intimate task.

Sometimes, despite best efforts, long-term breastfeeding is just not in the cards for some mamas. You've heard it said, "Breast is best." But when the poopy diaper hits the fan, fed is best!

My first child breastfed for five months. It never felt easy, as she was a very impatient eater who struggled to wait for the letdown of milk. (Once baby starts sucking, it still might take a minute before your body gets the message to let 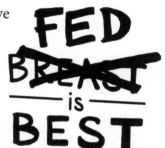 something out.) When my second child seemed to catch on to the technique right off the bat, I was thrilled, thinking she was destined for a perfect year of breastfeeding. However, after only three months, she decided we were done. What? Once you return to work and have to start pumping, keeping up enough supply for your baby can become an issue, as it did for me. In the end, both my kiddos were breastfed through their most vulnerable months but formula-fed for most of the first year of life. You'd never know the difference. They both kept growing fast and strong with very few episodes of illness.

The moral of the story is simple: Try your best to stick with breastfeeding as long as you can, but if it doesn't work out the way you had hoped, it doesn't make you a failure. It's just God's plan. He can use breastmilk or formula to help that baby grow and thrive!

Hormones and Emotions

Crying is normal, and it's okay. (I'm talking about you, not the baby.) You may cry for reasons that are obvious, or you may be laughing one minute and bursting into tears the next with no idea why. Just warn your husband to expect this and that long hugs and words of affirmation and encouragement will make it all better. Your hormones will be all over the map at times, so you might as well ride that tidal wave and embrace the emotional freedom of not having to explain yourself.

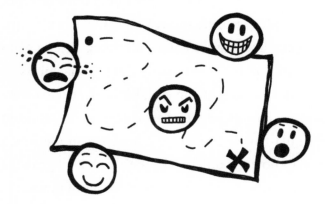

Part of the emotional roller coaster may include sadness. It might make no sense, and it might make you feel like a horrible person. Why would you feel *sad* when you've been so intensely blessed? This is supposed to be the happiest time in your entire life! Nonetheless, you may have moments where you just feel kind of sad. Don't worry, just let it happen. It's normal. Don't feel bad about it. Your brain may be processing things—or maybe it really has no good explanation. Your hormones are just trying to stabilize again. Talk to someone about it if you want; never be ashamed of it! And as always, let your almighty God and Savior comfort you through it. It will pass!

If you ever feel like you're sad more than you're happy, tell your OB/GYN. Postpartum depression is a real thing, and you can't get help if no one knows how you're feeling. Check out the Edinburgh Postnatal Depression Scale (you can find it online) to screen yourself if you feel you are struggling with this and might need help. This can help educate you on the symptoms to look for, but in the end you definitely need to consult your health care provider. If you do, don't be ashamed. It doesn't mean you don't love your child or that you're a bad mom. Quite the opposite, in fact. I would argue that it proves you love your child and that you're willing to do what it takes to be the best mama you can be! The sooner you seek help, the sooner you can get back to enjoying precious time with that baby of yours.

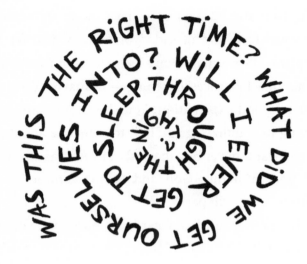

It's okay and totally normal to have mixed emotions about the realities of being a parent. All at once, you have to commit your life to another human being. Although this is a wonderful blessing, it can also leave you feeling overwhelmed from time to time. Dare I say, it can even make you second-guess from time to time. Was this really the right time? What did we get ourselves into? Is there any hope of going back to the way things were? There will be times when you just want some sleep. Or some quiet. Or a shower without worrying if the baby is crying. Or a simple date without a time limit. There will be times when you just want your body back. *Sister, it's okay.*

Don't hide these feelings—they don't make you a bad mom!

You may have feelings of loss and grief for the life you had before the baby or the person you were before you had this huge new responsibility. It doesn't mean you don't love your baby more than anything else on this earth.

Talk to a friend, your mom, or your husband about it. Cry about it if you want to. See if you can arrange an opportunity to revert to your pre-baby self for an hour or two. Have hubby take the baby while you go to the gym, or simply go for a walk with a friend. These types of short breaks are so powerful!

It's a positive and necessary thing to focus on yourself once in a while. Chances are you'll feel a lot better, and then you can redirect your focus to that sweet little blessing who turned your world upside down. These challenging times will be just memories before you know it, and you'll see it was all worth it.

Healing

Your body, including your pelvic floor, *will* heal. It's okay to feel sad and frustrated at the state of things for the first few days and weeks. Initial pelvic floor problems can be scary. Cut yourself some slack and remember that healing takes time.

I broke down in tears a few days after delivering my first baby. (I know, there were a lot of tears.) When I went to sit on the toilet, I realized I was already peeing and didn't even know it. I was mortified, having never felt so undignified in my life. I was worried it would be a long-term problem, but it never happened again. In fact, I think the sheer act of being a mom and rarely having the opportunity to use the bathroom is God's natural pelvic floor rehabilitation for postpartum incontinence.

Even if incontinence, pelvic pain, or some other issue persists, you have resources to help fix it. Just because you had a baby does not mean you are doomed to have embarrassing pelvic floor problems for the rest of your life.

As a physical therapist specializing in pelvic floor rehab, I would be doing you a disservice here if I did not mention that pelvic floor PT can do wonders in helping you regain normal pelvic floor function. Far too many women hold the misconception that incontinence, pelvic pain, or lower back pain are inevitable after having children, and that these are lifelong burdens they have to bear. This is not true!

The pelvic floor is a group of muscles, and just like any other part of the body, these muscles can have weakness, tightness, or asymmetries that can be corrected and retrained. If you have a persisting problem, talk to your OB/GYN about a referral to PT, making sure you seek a pelvic floor specialist. It will change your life.

It's normal to have a lot of bleeding after vaginal delivery, even after you leave the hospital. A good rule of thumb on when to let your doctor know is if you are soaking through a large pad within an hour. Keep an eye on it, but don't be surprised by anything less than that. It will slowly decrease week by week, and should be completely done by the time you follow up with your OB at six weeks postpartum.

It's a good idea to keep a supply of extra-large pads in your bathroom before baby arrives. (Husbands don't love going to the store to get that stuff.)

A noticeable increase in the amount of bleeding may be a sign that you are doing too much activity. For example, if, after four weeks, you have very little bleeding and then

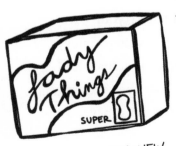

↖ EVEN MORE NEW BESTIES

start bleeding again after a four-mile walk, you might want to dial it back a notch. You've probably overworked your pelvic floor.

When is it safe to return to sex? If you're anything like me, that will be the *last* thing you'll want to think about after everything that happened down there. Don't worry, my friend. You will have sex again!

Go your own pace. Be patient with yourself and your healing, along with any emotional baggage you may have because of the fact that you just had a traumatic day in which you pushed a human being out of your body. Make sure to communicate with your husband about how you are feeling in regards to getting back to sex so he knows you're not avoiding him, but that you may just need some time. It may also help to warn him that you might need to be the one in control the first few times, to avoid additional pelvic floor muscle tension or pain.

Expect soreness in more than just your pelvic floor or abdomen. You may use muscles you never thought would be involved during the actual childbirth. (My biceps were so sore the week after my first daughter was born, I thought I must have torn them.) Without question though, you'll definitely be sore in the weeks (even months) that follow,

YOUR BODY is amazing AND SO ARE you!

simply from the postures you need to assume to take care of a completely helpless newborn.

I think I started getting carpal tunnel syndrome in one wrist from the way I held the baby, and my lower back and upper back definitely felt postural strains. Even my knees felt it, from all the deep squatting and kneeling I suddenly had to start doing to take care of my new baby.

Do your best to take care of yourself. I say do your best because this becomes surprisingly difficult to prioritize once you have a new, more delicate life to look after. See a massage therapist or a physical therapist if necessary; be proactive about posture as much as you can; take a few minutes to stretch where you need it, etc. Easier said than done—but try!

Download my free educational PDF's on postpartum postures to avoid and a postpartum exercise program to get a great start! You can find these on my website at www.kristenemilybehl.com.

In the weeks or months following delivery, your cute, firm, baby bump will be replaced with a squishy, loose, five-months-pregnant-sized bump. This. Is. Normal.

It's okay if you want to be proactive about strengthening your pelvic floor or restoring some abdominal tone, but resist that urge to rush yourself to break the record for fastest flat tummy or fastest weight loss after childbirth. Seriously, sweet friend. Mamas can be *so hard* on themselves.

The truth is, although you can return to pre-baby weight and get your abdominal function back without significant diastasis recti (persistent separation of your six-pack abs), your abdomen is never going to be exactly the same as it was before you got pregnant. Look at how much that abdomen has to stretch and loosen for baby. That post-baby bump will go away, but the firmness that you might be used to from your fitter pre-baby abdomen may never be quite as good as it was before. Your abdomen will probably look and feel smaller in the morning than in the evening or after a big meal, because when your abdominals are relaxed, the front wall of the abdominal cavity is stretchier than it used to be. It just is. No amount of abdominal training will fix that, because your abdominals are not turned on at all times. This is something no one will ever notice, besides you. Not even your husband.

There were times after both babies that I found myself staring into the bathroom mirror in my under-garments, agonizing over the new roundness in my abdomen that might always keep me from wearing the tight-fitting tops I used to wear. In one of those moments, Phil walked by and said, "Hey, you got your body back!" Bless that man! Even though it won't look exactly the same to you, you can still be confident that God will restore you to exactly how you are meant to be. Of course, do your best to treat that body right by giving it healthy food and exercise. From there, just be confident in how God made you!

Try not to fixate on how fast (or slow) the num-ber on the scale is decreasing each day. The first 10 or 15 pounds will drop off within the first few weeks (because you are minus one baby, one placenta, and a lot of fluid), but the rest will take three to six months, maybe more.

When you think about it, the postpartum period gives you the weight loss plan most people dream of. Even though you're trying to lose pregnancy weight, this should not keep you from eating as much as you want at dinner. You need to be nourished so baby can be nourished. It takes a lot of calories to constantly produce breastmilk.

God will take care of you. Be smart, be healthy, but do not worry. Do not stress out about losing weight in those first few months. It will come. And remember the tiger stripes? The changes to your body that you can't control are a badge of honor, and a reminder that you've had the blessing of becoming a mama!

There is one simple way you can help yourself stay healthy after having your baby. Drink a *lot* of water! And then drink more water! Just like during pregnancy, your body needs incredible amounts of hydration in order to produce breastmilk and to keep your own systems working and healing.

I was terrible at remembering to drink water, and I often paid for it with chronic headaches and lightheadedness. Once I even passed out briefly after I stood up too fast, broke a nightlight on the way down, and really freaked out my husband. Seriously, drink more water! I also developed an intense hatred of bowel movements. When your pelvic floor is trying to heal, you do not want to be straining or dealing with hard stools. Trust me on this one. Hydrate, woman!

Finally, let's not forget about mental and emotional healing. It might take some time for you to mentally process what your body just went through. Having a baby is a beautiful, happy occasion, but don't forget that there is very real trauma for the one who has to push that baby out. It will help to talk to someone about what you just endured. Call your mom or another mama friend who has been through it too.

The first night we brought our daughter home, I found myself in tears around 7:00 p.m. with no idea why. The baby was sleeping peacefully in her room, the kitchen was clean because my awesome husband just tidied it up while I was napping, yet there I was sobbing with no explanation. Phil hugged me, told me it was okay, and encouraged me to call my mom. She was at my house within the hour, and all she did was listen while I recounted my whole birth story and how it made me feel. I felt so much better after that.

I think once I finally had a moment to settle into my home again and tried to relax, that's when my brain had the chance to relive it all, to process the epic day that we had looked forward to in mystery for so long. As we tried to get back to normal in our home, my brain just couldn't deny the feeling that I *wasn't* quite the same as when I last left the house. Childbirth changed me. Not necessarily in a way most people would notice, but it changed the way I felt, the way I saw myself, and the way I thought about my body. It was a huge ordeal, mentally, physically, and emotionally.

Let yourself process however you need to, and remember how strong you are with the help of your amazing Creator!

Be patient with your body as it works in hyperdrive to supply breastmilk, drop the pregnancy weight, regain strength, stabilize hormones, heal, and keep itself going on very little sleep. Seriously, mama, give yourself some credit!

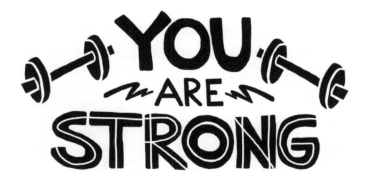

Postpartum Exercise

I have compiled a handy-dandy PDF that you can download free from my website at www.kristenemilybehl.com. As a pelvic floor rehabilitation specialist, I wanted to supply you with some valuable education and specific exercises to help you regain strength in all the areas that are typically weakened during pregnancy and childbirth. In the document, you can learn what your core actually is, how your pelvic floor is designed to function, and a simple exercise program to train those muscles and prevent problems. You can self-progress through the program at your own pace, as your body tolerates. I recommend printing it out now and keeping it handy for after baby arrives, when you're ready to use it.

Take it slow and gentle. Doing too much physical activity too soon can create new problems.

Give your body time to heal before demanding too much from yourself. The ligaments throughout your whole body will stay lax as long as you are breastfeeding (because of the hormones involved), which means your joints won't be as stable as you're used to during that time. This makes them prone to injury or chronic pain if you over stress them.

You should not be doing anything high-impact before six weeks postpartum. Even if you feel stellar, doing things like jogging or jumping jacks are inflicting lots of stress on weak core muscles and stretched-out ligaments. It's possible to do more harm than good.

The pelvic floor is a high-endurance group of muscles. Walking doesn't seem that strenuous, but when you just had a baby, that's asking those weak muscles to do a lot of stabilizing and supporting.

Even six weeks after my first delivery, I only tolerated walking one to two miles before I felt like my abdominal organs might fall out, as my pelvic floor muscles fatigued. But by training slowly, I was able to jog a 5K with a stroller at 12 weeks without pain or any negative physical repercussions. The key is to listen to your healing body. It's a positive thing to make goals for yourself, but you have to have realistic expectations to achieve them and be willing to modify if your body says no.

Ease into it; slowly work your way back to your normal. It doesn't mean you're weak. It means you're smart.

Relationship Maintenance After Baby Arrives

After you have the baby, you will be out of commission (as far as your husband is concerned) for at least a few weeks. Technically you should wait six weeks until you see your OB again, but some people feel comfortable resuming sex before that. On the contrary, even when the OB gives you the go-ahead after six weeks, you might still have some hesitation, as things might still feel sore or traumatized to some extent.

Take it slow, do it when you feel ready, but definitely have a conversation about it with your husband even before you have the baby. Let him know what to expect—or even that you don't know what to expect from yourself. Let him know you will need his patience and understanding, and that he may need to use a different love language for a little while. Explain that it's not personal, and it's not that you don't *want* to have sex with him again. It's just that it can be a little scary, especially if you had any significant tearing or other factors that can make healing (physically or mentally) a longer process.

Whenever you do feel ready to get back at it, don't forget that it's possible to get pregnant even if you are exclusively breastfeeding. Just ask my ultrasound tech, who had two babies ten months apart! Use this information as you will.

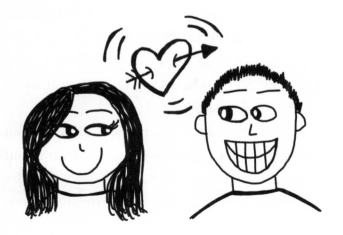

Don't be surprised if sex is really uncomfortable or even hurts the first several times. This short-term discomfort is normal. Think about it. Aside from pregnancy, if you had any kind of significant physical trauma six weeks ago—broken bone, muscle tear, surgery—your body isn't going to like being provoked there. No matter how delivery goes for you, it's traumatic for your pelvis! All of your lower abdominal contents are trying to find their place again after a very sudden change in the size of your uterus. In the event of a vaginal delivery, your vaginal walls just had an intense encounter with your baby's giant head. Cut yourself some slack! Things are going to look and feel—maybe even sound—a little different. But with patience and time, it will get better.

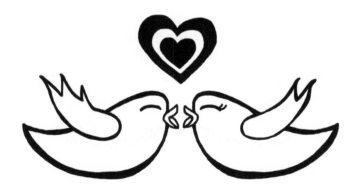

It may be wise to buy some high-quality lubricant that's water-based and free of chemicals that may irritate the sensitive vaginal walls. Your OB can probably recommend a brand. Breastfeeding can cause dryness, even if you've never had that problem before. Lube will eliminate this issue and make it a much more comfortable experience.

My best recommendation is to ask your husband to let you lead. If you can be in control of speed and movement the first several times you have sex again, you'll be able to avoid unintentionally traumatizing (for lack of a better word) the pelvic floor even more and making the problem worse. You want those muscles to relax. You want to retrain them to be okay with letting something in.

Remember, once you do feel ready for sex again, there will still be barriers that may not have existed before. The combination of low energy and terrible sleep has the potential to diminish your sex life. This is really hard on a marriage, especially when the husband isn't dealing with the physical issues that his wife has after baby is born. You are always in charge of how you choose to spend the limited energy you have, but make sure to prioritize your sex life in some way. This is one of the biggest ways you can keep your bond with your husband super strong through these crazy times.

Your husband might be feeling replaced after baby is born. His time with you will be temporarily replaced with him picking up slack for you while you catch another much-needed nap, or with him encouraging you in feeding the new life that now exists in your home.

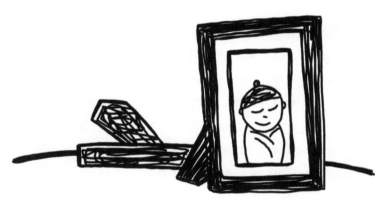

Every so often, for no apparent reason, put that sweet little baby down and hug your hubby. Remind him that he is still your favorite adult human.

Similarly, a frequent debacle you may find yourself in is how to spend your time when baby is napping. You can A) Take care of yourself, B) Take care of your husband (as in quality time), or C) Take care of your house. This tug-of-war inside you is real, and there's no black and white answer. Just recognize the tug-of-war, embrace the blessings

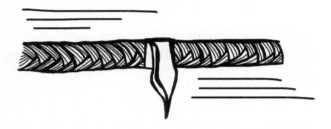

that put you in this situation, and make the decision one instance at a time.

It also wouldn't hurt to confide in your husband about this. Let him know you feel pulled in several directions with very limited time and energy, and that this will persist pretty much until baby lets you sleep more normal hours at night. Help him sympathize and understand how you feel. It might decrease some of the stress or guilt in the times you don't choose him.

Acknowledge that this is hard for him too. He may not be the one feeding at all hours of the night or dealing with physical healing like you are, but he is going through a huge life change just like you are, and he's probably not getting as much sleep as usual either. He's trying to figure out his new roles, too.

A trap that I often find myself falling into is the "Who's working harder?" game.

It's not really a game. It's a horrible mental tally of which spouse is giving more. When you feel like you are giving absolutely everything you have and being more selfless than you ever thought possible, it's hard *not* to play this game. But if/when you feel this happening, step back and consider all the things your husband has been doing for baby or for you—things he has taken care of financially or physically around the house. Things that you couldn't do or didn't have time to do. Focus on the wonderful things he does. If you are still feeling like there is more you need from him, bring it up to him humbly, and be specific.

Here are some practical ways to keep your marriage as healthy as possible during the postpartum period:

+ Schedule a one or two-hour date. (You can get home in time to feed the baby.) Have a trusted sitter come over while you're gone. Family works best if that's an option for you. Otherwise, consider another mom from church, a friend who knows her way around a diaper, etc. You *must* trust this person—it will make your date much more relaxing. It's not easy leaving baby for the first time, even for just a couple of hours, so having a sitter you are confident with can make all the difference in the enjoyment of your special date.

+ Go out for dinner. It doesn't have to be fancy!

+ Take a long walk. Hold hands, kiss on a park bench, talk about your feelings, compliment each other.

+ I don't recommend a movie unless it's something both of you are dying to see and you know it will be a good way to bond. This time should be focused on your relationship—being together and talking, giving each other the attention that has been temporarily stolen by that cute little baby. And let's be honest, you'd just fall asleep at a movie.

+ Go to the gym and work out together. You won't be able to do anything too strenuous yet, but you'll feel amazing even after a walk or elliptical at your tolerated pace.

+ Surprise your husband with a gift of gratitude—a small token that you know he'll appreciate, to show him how much you love him for all the help and encouragement he has given you.

+ Give him your blessing for a guilt-free night out with his friends. Try to have a friend or family member come to hang out with you if you feel this would make things really hard for you.

+ Tell him if there is something that would make your day.
+ Ask him what *he* needs.
+ Remember that your hormones might be a little hard for him to keep up with, and try to communicate clearly.

FINDING NEW DEPTHS OF SELFLESS LOVE

You are doing so great, pregnant little mama. Amazing. Your baby has no idea the blessings that are coming; how beautiful life is going to be; how much love you have to give. But he or she will find out soon!

You'll be amazed at the level of selflessness you can access once you become a mom. It's not easy to be this selfless *all* the time. It's a big change at first, especially because most of that selflessness is only seen by someone too tiny to verbalize appreciation for it.

Seriously, this can really get to you!

Even your husband, as wonderful as he will be during this time, probably won't understand everything you do behind the scenes, both now and in the years to come. There will come a day when you realize how much you took for granted simple plea-sures like eating food while it's still hot, or making it through the whole meal without needing to leave the table to get something for someone else, or not waking up to the sound of crying.

When you feel overwhelmed by your unceas-ing (and often under-appreciated) caregiving role, remember how hard you prayed for this. Remember the ways God has satisfied your long-ings with this child. Recognize the pure blessing it is to have these problems, because it means that you are mama to a healthy child and wife to an amazing man.

There are *so* many amazing, hilarious, beautiful ways this baby is going to enhance your life, your marriage, and your purpose. There are *so* many things to savor about the postpartum period. I know I didn't spend a lot of time talking about the more positive aspects of it, but that's because you already know them. They are the parts everyone talks about! As I close this letter, I want to focus on these things, too.

Every time you're breastfeeding in the middle of the night and all you want to do is go back to bed, think instead of how short a time you get to hold that baby before he or she grows into a wild child.

Every time you sigh in frustration that yet another outfit has been spit up on, think instead about that sweet baby breath and the smell of baby hair as you snuggle close in a fresh new outfit.

Savor those sweet, tiny fingers against your face, the softest skin you'll ever feel.

Soak in each precious, heart-melting giggle and coo; enjoy every sound of your baby's voice before you have the need to discipline.

Totally own that pride, that new identity you feel every time you take baby out in public or to see friends and family.

Revel in the excitement of each new skill your child learns at each phase of growth, as you get to experience each one as a mama for the very first time.

Watch that precious miracle sleep, with your husband's arms wrapped around you. Thank God for this perfect plan He has orchestrated for your life. Wonder together who the Lord will shape this child to be.

In all the craziness of the postpartum time, these are truly the moments that you'll remember and cherish for the rest of your days. These are the things that will give you nostalgia when that little baby is running off to kindergarten or graduating from high school or getting married.

It's all so worth it

It's all *so* worth it!

You're going to rock this, mama. Absolutely, without question.

Here's a hug for you!

Love, Kristen

> "Jesus Christ is the same
> yesterday, today, and forever."
> —Hebrews 13:8

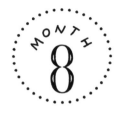

Final Encouragement

My dear, radiant, pregnant friend,

THIS IS, AS THEY SAY, THE FINAL COUNT-
down! You have reached month eight of your
nine-month journey through pregnancy.

Can you *believe* it?

It feels like just yesterday you were first sharing
the news, bursting at the seams with excitement.
Here we are today, knowing that only a few short
weeks stand between you and holding that real,

YOU'RE ALMOST THERE!

warm, snuggly baby in your arms. In just a few weeks, you'll get your first glance at that precious face.

You'll get to feel teeny tiny fingers wrap around one of yours.

You'll get to melt into that brand new baby skin against your chest and breathe in that sweet new baby smell that is unlike anything else in the world.

You'll get to physically see and touch that miraculous blend of you and your husband and marvel at how this beautiful being came into existence.

You'll get to watch your husband be a daddy who'll cradle and stare at his most precious blessing in a way you've never seen before.

Tissue break...long sigh...

Okay, where was I?

In a few short weeks, you'll get to look into your child's eyes and wonder, "Who has God designed you to be? What adventures will you have? What qualities did God give you that make you who you are? What will you excel at, and how will you fail? (There will be failures, of course, and that's a good thing!) What kind of trouble will you get into?

What depths of sweetness and love will you possess? What will you be when you grow up? What will you teach me? How many grandbabies will you make me?"

Whoa, Bessy, back this baby bus up! Let's not get ahead of ourselves.

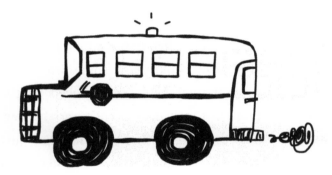

The best part about all this dreaming and wondering is that you're almost there! Can you feel—or even see—those little kicks, letting you know that baby is getting strong and ready to meet you? I wish your baby could see the beautiful mama who's been waiting and the intense comfort you'll provide. This child is so blessed to have you.

In this final pre-baby letter, I want you to simply pause in the silence and stillness of your home.

Take a long, cleansing breath. Seriously, do it.

Hear the quiet.

Be in this moment.

Savor this feeling of wonder, mystery, and anticipation.

Be deeply encouraged by what I am about to say.

FINAL ENCOURAGEMENT

An awful lot of information has been thrown your way since you started spreading the news of your pregnancy. There are some important truths that sometimes get overshadowed by the well-meaning "Just wait until..." lecturers in your life. You know, the people who have a hard time just offering a friendly, "Congratulations! I'm so excited for you!" Instead, they like to point out during your one-minute conversations all the ways you aren't prepared for this or the struggles they are sure you've never heard are coming.

I'm sure these people just aren't thinking through how you're feeling. They might have a subconscious need to demonstrate

PIECE of CAKE? HA!

their own expertise on the subject, or they'd like to be applauded for mastering their own pregnancies or parenting experiences. I mean, it is a feat to be sure, and good for them! Shouldn't they know, then, that a new mom could use encouragement rather than pessimism? Every pregnant woman knows that becoming a mom is no cake walk. No one has to tell her that—especially in a way that feels even the least bit belittling.

Instead, here in the peace and comfort of your home, try to reflect on the positivity of the over-shadowed truths of becoming a mama.

TRUTH #1: You can do this.

Whether it's being a mom in general, labor and delivery, or simply surviving another night of discomfort with that giant baby belly—*you can do this*! I promise! It feels like such a huge change coming, and of course it is. You've dealt with change before, and God has always led you through it. He uses changes and challenges to shape you into a more

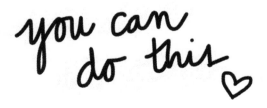

beautiful work of art than you were before.

Think of Mary, the mother of Jesus. How terrified she must have felt, having a baby in that day and age, under suspicious circumstances to the outside observer. How scary it must have been, not having the expertise of any doctor—only her carpenter husband. How emotionally draining it must have been to not have the support of most of the people in her life. Think of the pressure she must have felt to be a great mama to the Son of God! We know she wasn't perfect. Remember when she lost track of him for three days during their journey home from the Passover festival when he was only 12 years old?

Not her proudest moment, probably.

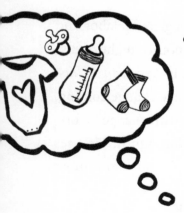

Imagine how much that child changed her. Made her better. Reinforced her faith. Imagine her peace, feeling God beside her when she otherwise might have felt alone.

He is beside you, too, just like He was for Mary. He is going to make you better and stronger through this journey. He will make you more capable of love and selflessness. You will identify weaknesses and strengths within yourself you never noticed before. Lean on Him, trust in Him, and know that He has prepared you fully for this greatest of earthly blessings.

The gravity of motherhood is more daunting than anything you've ever done or ever will do. God has entrusted you with His precious little lamb, both physically and spiritually. I know it will make all those self-doubts rise to the surface. I know there will be times that you'll feel inadequate and unprepared. In the end, God will not fail you. He has equipped you with what you need to succeed. With His help, you can do this!

TRUTH #2: You are beautiful.

Motherhood is full of really glamorous moments: standing all dressed up in front of church and beaming as the Holy Spirit works faith in your new baby's heart through the sacrament of Holy Baptism; pushing that baby in the jogger while you walk or run behind, with

you are beautiful ♡

all the passers-by nodding in recognition of the impressiveness of your post-baby energy; smiling and laughing with your baby as you share Hallmark moments together on the sunlit living room carpet.

These are coming, and these are awesome!

But sometimes, perhaps much more often than it should, motherhood can make you feel anything but glamorous. When you feel this way, I want you to shrug your shoulders and say, "Oh well. At least I know I'm normal!" and just keep being you.

I know we've covered this before, but it's something you can never hear enough. You are *beautiful*, my friend. The exhaustion and lack of showering that comes with new mama territory tends to bring other adjectives to mind first—things like *old*, *tired*, *haggard*—because we think we look how we feel, and we certainly don't always feel beautiful.

Let me share a story with you:

Before I had my own kids, I was standing in the checkout line at Aldi after work one day. I watched in awe as a young woman ahead of me juggled three small children by herself—one in the front seat of the cart, one on the ground next to the cart, and one strapped into a carrier on her back. She was on high alert, focused on unloading the groceries from her cart to the conveyor belt while also keeping an eye on the two kids in front of her. Meanwhile, the one on her back had discovered that he could reach the products for sale in the checkout aisle whenever mama stood upright. It was a hilarious little cycle of grabbing a handful of granola bars from the aisle and dropping them into the cart in rhythm with mom's unloading. He was having a blast.

When his mama finally noticed the mischief, it became a whole new hysterical scene. Mom would take the new granola bars out of the cart and place them back on the rack, while clever kiddo would grab a new handful of something else from further down the aisle and throw it into the cart. The cycle continued for 20 seconds or so until that sweet little mama finally found a position where the tot couldn't reach the products, which took some finagling between the cart and the kid on the ground.

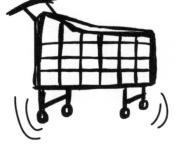

All the while, although she was likely feeling frustrated, exhausted, awkward, and embarrassed, the only thought I had was how incredible she was. She was beautiful. No make-up, hair in a messy bun, yoga pants and a T-shirt, covered in groceries and children, and clearly struggling. I didn't have kids yet at that point, so I can't even say I could empathize with her or really understand how she felt. All I know is, as an unbiased third-party observer, to me that lady was awesome and beautiful.

That's how people will see you, because that's how you truly are. Beautiful. Even if others only know a fraction of what you're going through, they can still see the beauty of a mother caring for her child. They don't care how greasy your hair is, or that your socks don't match, or that your stomach isn't flat. They see a mama giving of herself for the love of her child, taking care of her family, and that is *honestly* the most radiant sight!

It's amazing how many smiles you'll get from complete strangers, simply because they see you being a mom. You may be stewing over a frustrating moment when a stranger walks by and says, "Aw, this just makes my day!" Suddenly you are brought back to the reality that you and your child and the interactions you share are just...so... beautiful. Then you might cry. In public. And guess what? You're still beautiful!

TRUTH #3: You are loved.

My mom's birthday is the day after mine. She always joked (with some truth behind it) that everyone forgot about her birthday as soon as I was born. It sounds harsh, but let's face it—we make a way bigger deal out of kid birthdays than parent birthdays. (You little sweetheart, I know what you're thinking. Don't worry, my mom's birthday was never actually forgotten.)

My point is only that once a baby joins your family, it might feel at times like all the love from others that used to be directed at you is suddenly directed at the baby. This is not a bad thing, of course. However, as you keep sacrificing and giving of yourself for this baby that is so loved, supported, and cared about, your own needs might feel neglected from time to time.

This is your friendly reminder that you are dearly loved, my friend. Even when everything seems to revolve around baby, you are still surrounded by people who care deeply for *you*. You have so much value, and you always will, through every season of life.

Look at these words:

"For you created my inmost being;
You knit me together in my mother's womb.
I praise you because I am fearfully and
wonderfully made;
Your works are wonderful,
I know that full well." —Psalm 139:13-14

Having a baby does not transfer this truth from you to the baby—it's true of both of you. You are still a precious work of God's design. You are just as beautiful to Him today (and to the rest of your loved ones) as the day you were born, when everyone ooh'ed and aah'ed over the miracle that is you.

You're still that miracle.

Most importantly, your Heavenly Father thinks you are valuable and lovable enough that He gave up His own Son in your place—despite your sinfulness and your failures. Jesus thought you were valuable enough to willingly suffer hell and die so that you can spend eternity in heaven with Him.

That's an awful lot of love, and it will never, ever fade away as the seasons of your life change.

If you're having a moment where you aren't feeling the love you need, seek Jesus in His Word, tell your husband you could use a big hug, and call your mama or your best friend. They'll quickly remind you how loved you are.

TRUTH #4: God chose YOU.

The Bible is jam-packed with scenarios where God selects a seemingly unfit or unremarkable person to do extraordinary things for His glory. When He needed a soldier to defeat the giant

God chose you ♡

Goliath and rescue His people from battle, He chose a teenage shepherd named David who had never fought a battle in his life. He also chose David to be one of His most beloved kings despite some egregious sins. When God needed a man to boldly spread His gospel message across nations, He picked Paul, who had previously been responsible for the horrifying persecution of God's people. These are remarkable demonstrations of how well God knows His children, how masterfully He has crafted them, and how powerfully He can use them to make a difference.

For this baby's mama, God chose YOU. He doesn't make mistakes. He knows you just like He knew David and Paul. He's been cultivating your purpose from the moment of your conception. He's been leading you forward in fulfillment of that purpose day by day. It doesn't mean the journey will be easy, but it will be exactly as He planned it. God sees your strengths and weaknesses, and He decided that this child is perfect for no one but you.

TRUTH #5: You chose life.

You have already protected your little one through the most vulnerable and fragile phase of life. You did everything in your power to nourish, comfort, and love baby even before birth. To you and me it seems like a given, but sadly we know that in today's world, conception of a child does not guarantee that the child will be wanted or taken care of.

you chose life ♡

You chose life. You chose life for your child over convenience for yourself. You chose a lifelong commitment of self-sacrifice and unconditional love. You chose to accept all the unpleasantries and all the unknowns, understanding that abundant joy will be remembered most. You chose to place your life, your baby's life, your marriage, your body, your future, all in God's hands by guarding and protecting the precious new life that He has blessed you with. This makes your Heavenly Father very happy! This is what He desires from the mama He chose.

You are already rocking it!

you are NOT alone ♡

TRUTH #6: You are not alone.

You are intensely loved by your husband, your Savior, your family and your friends. You are never alone in this journey.

When you feel joy, you will not be alone.

When you feel sadness, you will not be alone.

When you feel excitement, you will not be alone.

When you feel overwhelmed, you will not be alone.

When you rejoice, or when you struggle, you will not be alone.

When you feel clueless, you are SO not alone!

When you feel victorious or defeated, you will not be alone.

Use the people God has placed around you to support you, not only during this time of pregnancy, but in all the days that follow. Mama of a newborn, toddler, middle-schooler, teenager, and all at once you're an empty-nester. Life is full of transitions, and you'll be adapting to a game where the rules always change. The team members on your bench may sub in and out depending on the phase of life in which each person may best support you, but in the end they are all players in your championship saga. Lean on them, love them, and feel the strength God offers through them. You, of course, are a member of their teams too, and they will surely lean on you from time to time as well. Soak in all the energy you can absorb from those cheering you on, and from those who are in the struggle right there with you. This is the purpose of friendships, marriage, and family.

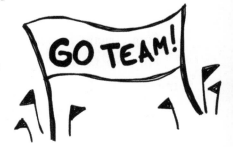

Sister, you are almost there! Your joy and excitement is rejuvenating to those who see you and know you. The happiness in your soul is being absorbed by that precious new life growing closer and closer to meeting you.

Can you imagine what it will be like to stare straight into the eyes of your new baby? Can you fathom how your heart will feel as you lose yourself in their depths?

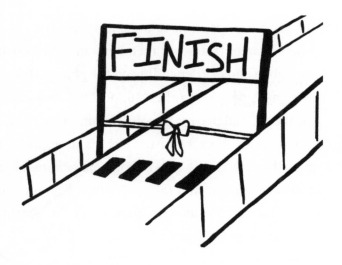

Soon, friend. So soon!

For now, take another deep breath as you savor the silence of your home. Enjoy every daydream about what it will be like to have this baby. Reflect on your blessings thus far on your journey of life, and take time to thank God for where He's brought you. Spend some time talking to Him, out loud or in your mind. Tell Him your excitement, your fears, your hopes, your doubts. Go to His Word to hear His encouragement and reassurance:

> "I sought the Lord, and he answered me; he delivered me from all my fears. Those who look to him are radiant; their faces are never covered with shame." —Psalm 34:4-5

"Your hands made me and formed me; give me understanding to learn your commands. May those who fear you rejoice when they see me, for I have put my hope in your word." —Psalm 119:73-74

"Clap your hands, all you nations; shout to God with cries of joy. How awesome is the Lord Most High, the great King over all the earth!" —Psalm 47:1-2

"Delight yourself in the Lord and he will give you the desires of your heart. Commit your way to the Lord; trust in him and he will do this: He will make your righteousness shine like the dawn." —Psalm 37:4-6

"So I say to you: Ask and it will be given to you; seek and you will find; knock and the door will be opened to you. For everyone who asks receives; he who seeks finds; and to him who knocks, the door will be opened. Which of you fathers, if your son asks for a fish, will give him a snake instead? Or if he asks for an egg, will give him a scorpion? If you then, though you are evil, know how to give good gifts to your children, how much more will

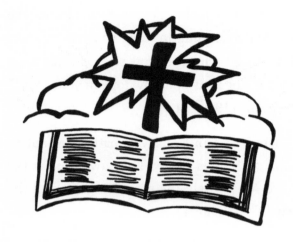

your Father in heaven give the Holy Spirit to those who ask him!" —Luke 11:9-13

"Rejoice in the Lord always, I will say it again: Rejoice! Let your gentleness be evident to all. The Lord is near. Do not be anxious about anything, but in everything, by prayer and petition, with thanksgiving, present your requests to God. And the peace of God, which transcends all understanding, will guard your hearts and minds in Christ Jesus." —Philippians 4:4-7

You've got this, my friend! So many prayers are headed up to heaven on your behalf. God is taking care of both of you, and He will bring you through this next month with all the strength and confidence you need. Keep trusting Him, as you have to this point. Before you know it, you'll be sitting in the hospital with your child in your arms—a bona fide mama! And you will be great. There's not a doubt in my mind.

Your next letter, Month Nine, is not to be read until you are in the hospital, baby and all. My vision is that you'll be able to find some quiet time to read it—perhaps when daddy and baby are sleeping peacefully while joy and adrenaline keep you awake.

Love you so much, dear friend! I am *so excited* for what's just around the corner for you!

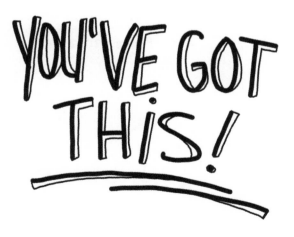

Rest up and enjoy this time with your main man!
Love, Kristen

"My soul
finds rest in God
alone; my salvation
comes from him. He
alone is my rock and my
salvation; he is my fortress,
I will not be shaken."
—Psalm 62:1-2

Congratulations!

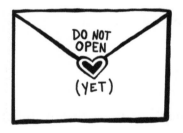

Bring in your maternity bag. DO NOT READ until you're in the hospital after baby is born!

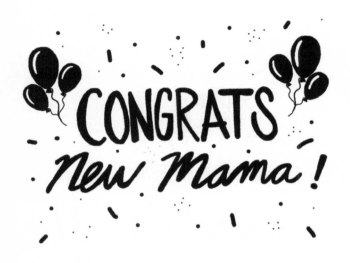

Dear sweet new mama,

I'M VISUALIZING THE SETTING YOU ARE in as I write this, envisioning that the ambiance is close enough to mine that it might feel like I could be right there with you. I'm on a comfy couch in my basement, snuggled under a blanket, crickets and night bugs chirping outside, kiddos peacefully sleeping upstairs. It's quiet. I picture that it's quiet in your moment too. I imagine you resting in your hospital bed, lights dimmed, hubby finally getting some rest on the couch beside you. You finally have a moment to breathe and reflect. You can finally begin to process what you just went through.

Your baby is sleeping, wrapped up tight in a blanket. *Your baby.*

My friend…you just had a *baby*! Congratulations!

I hope you can feel my long-distance embrace, stretching across the Wisconsin farmland and all the space between us to squeeze you in my arms and whisper, "You did it, girl. You really did it. Smile your beautiful smile. It's over. You did it."

I'm so proud of you! I hope you're proud of yourself. You absolutely should be. God gave you everything you needed, just like you prayed for and just like He promised. He has brought you to this place right now where you can glance over to the bassinet that holds your long-awaited, beautiful baby and rejoice in the mystery that has just been revealed to you.

The child you prayed for is *finally* here. The child that has made you a mama.

You hear that? You're a *mom*!

How long have you dreamed of this moment? Is it like you always imagined it would be?

How are you feeling? Is your adrenaline still pumping? Could you sleep if you tried? Are you completely exhausted? Have you had a restful nap yet since it all happened?

What emotions are racing through your heart in this moment?

Treasure These Moments

Pause. Breathe in, breathe out. Close your eyes, and savor.

"But Mary treasured up all these things and pondered them in her heart." —Luke 2:19

Treasure up all these things, my friend. Ponder them in your heart.

What is your child's name? How did it feel to finally say it out loud? The moment you finally saw the adorable face that will forever give it life, did it just fit?

How did your husband do? Do you feel so proud of the man he is? Did you feel his support like never before? Did he astonish you as you watched him become Daddy before your eyes? Take this time to reflect back on these sweet snippets that were hard to spend enough time with in the moment, but that you want to cherish and remember for all of your days.

Look at your hus-
band now, and
consider all that he did
to show you love on this
life-changing day. God
gave him the strength
and wisdom he needed
as well. Did he come
through for you or what?
This has likely been
one of the scariest and
most intense moments
of his life, but somehow God
held him steadfast to be a solid rock for you. He continues to be the man of your dreams that you were so smitten with on your wedding day.

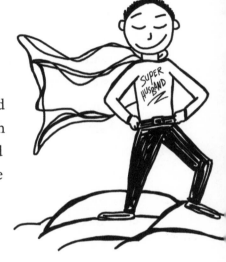

I'm excited for you to keep talking to each other about the experience you endured together. I'm excited for you to recognize and feel that incredible bond that you share because of it. I'm excited for you to hear about the day from his perspective. Knowing the details through each other's eyes will add to the specialness of every step (not to mention your husband probably has a much clearer memory of things you were too focused to notice at the time). You are one, after all.

I'm excited for you to relive this day over and over as you tell your birth story to family and friends, with the calmness and comfort that you did it. Instead of a mystery, it's now a memory.

I hope it was as positive an experience as delivering a baby can be. Did everything go according to plan?

What surprised you?

What was different than you expected?

Did you conquer your fears and achieve all your personal goals, or did God have a different plan for you?

Please be kind to yourself, sweet mama. Do not fall prey to the monster of comparison. Your

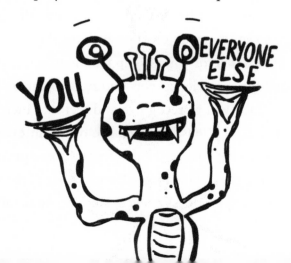

delivery experience is uniquely yours. However God designed it—whether smooth or disappointingly traumatic—it's *your* story. It's okay to let yourself feel one way or another as your mind processes what you've been through. I'm guessing even if things went pretty well, you're still feeling traumatized at some level. It's okay. Write it down, talk it out, find some way to acknowledge it, and start moving forward. Then focus on these next questions, and consider them over and over and over again:

How did it feel, the moment you knew your baby was finally on the outside? When you *finally* felt that tiny, soft weight against your skin? When you heard that newborn cry for the first time? The very moment your eyes saw a miracle?

Let your mind dwell on this, and store it in your heart forever.

How did it feel to try breastfeeding for the first time? I hope it went fantastic and felt natural and easy. Even if it didn't, you're still doing amazing by trying the best you can. Remember, it's a learning process for both of you, and everything is going to be okay. Really, it is. Your baby is going to be fed one way or another. God is taking care of this child. It's going to be okay.

Speaking of breastfeeding, how crazy is it—the speed at which you no longer care if everyone in the room sees you naked? Kind of hilarious, isn't it? It probably makes your husband way more uncomfortable than you.

How impressed are you with your medical team, not just during the process of labor and delivery, but in your care afterward? As you have seen, the job they do is far less than glamorous, but they are right there with you, never making you feel bad about cleaning up your messes. They are so giving and so kind. I'm sure they love having grateful, respectful, lovely patients like you!

How exhilarating was it to finally hear those all-important birth stats—pounds and ounces, inches, date and time—that are now ingrained in

hello my name is...

_____

_____ lbs _____ oz _____ ins

born ____/____/____

@ _____ AM/PM

your brain forever as the first details that defined your child?

Are you excited to get to know your baby more and more every day? To add to the list of defining qualities things like sleeping habits and feeding habits, things that provoke laughter and tears, personality?

Savor this feeling of unknown, of anticipation, of joy.

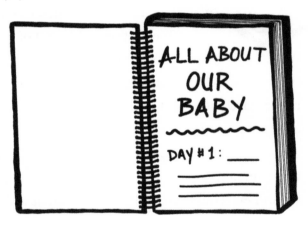

Look at your baby and marvel at this miracle of creation—how your Father in heaven formed, protected, and loves His precious new child.

When you feel that tiny heart beating so fast, can you feel the Holy Spirit working there? Can you hear the presence of Jesus whispering in that little ear, "Do not fear, for I have redeemed you;

I have summoned you by name; you are mine."
(Isaiah 43:1). Your baby, by the power of the Holy
Spirit and the washing away of his sinful nature in
baptism, has saving faith
in Jesus. Your baby
is safe, loved, and
most importantly,
saved.

Thank God for
this greatest news of all.
Feel the warm blanket of love
and protection in which Christ
envelops your little family this day. Let
it never leave your spirit as you begin the beautiful
journey of raising your child.

I hope you are resting comfortably without
much pain, and I hope you are enjoying those ice
pack undies. (Unless you had a C-section, in which
case, enjoy undies without ice packs.)

You get to move forward now. Delivery is complete. Page turn. Next chapter.

Are you *so excited* to see what comes next? I am!

You are going to be great, new mama. Enjoy
every moment of this incredibly special time. Have
no shame in taking ridiculous quantities of photos

and videos. Give that baby—and your amazing husband—so many hugs and kisses.

You are so loved, my amazing friend. I pray that Christ guides you from the very center of your heart, in every joy and every struggle, and that your child sees and feels this every day.

My heart is so happy when I think of you!

God bless you!

Love, Kristen

"Fix these words of mine in your hearts and minds; tie them as symbols on your hands and bind them on your foreheads. Teach them to your children, talking about them when you sit at home and when you walk along the road, when you lie down and when you get up. Write them on the doorframes of your houses and on your gates."

—Deuteronomy 11:18–20

A Letter to Yourself

A PLACE TO WRITE YOUR THOUGHTS

*I*T'S YOUR TURN NOW, NEW MAMA. WRITE down your own thoughts to help you process everything you just went through. Let yourself relive delivery day, and jot down every detail you never want to forget.

Hey, New Mama!

WANT MORE FRIENDLY INSIGHT AND encouragement as you enter the postpartum journey?

Download your FREE copy of my "Pelvic Floor and Core Exercise Program" and "Postpartum Postures" at www.KristenEmilyBehl.com to make sure you are taking care of YOU.

Then, check out the next book in the series, "Letters to the New Mama," coming soon!

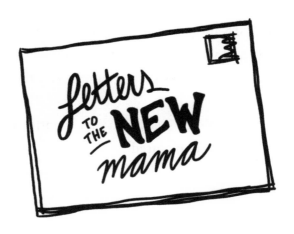

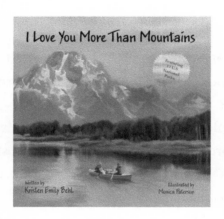

I Love You More Than Mountains

Immerse your children in the beauty and wonder of the U.S. National Parks. Help them comprehend how big and wide, how tall and deep your love for them will always be. These are memories they will never forget!

As you explore, see if you can identify which national parks are pictured!

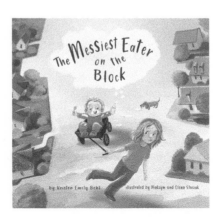

The Messiest Eater on the Block

A frustrated older sister tells her perspective of a little brother with such poor table manners that unwanted dinner guests begin showing up at the door. Get ready to make silly sounds and use your imagination as the young messy eaters in your family learn that they are loved despite—or because of—the messes.

Book 1 of the "On the Block" Series

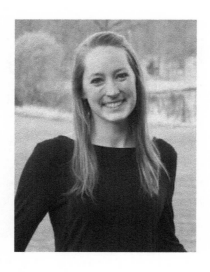

HELLO FROM ME TO YOU!

I am so thankful for you! I want to know who you are. Please shoot me an email at connect@kristenemilybehl.com to help me get to know you. Who are you? Where are you as you read these letters? What does your pregnancy or postpartum journey look like? I love to hear from readers and find out how I can better serve you!

Here's a little more about me:

I live out in the country in friendly Wisconsin, USA with my husband, Phil. We have two beautiful daughters who are 19 months apart. They are doing their best to teach us how to be good parents. We enjoy fostering a love for travel and the outdoors in our girls through cross-country road trips, off-roading, hiking, and wildlife viewing whenever we get the chance. We cheer for the Green Bay Packers, sing off-key in church, and cherish our amazing families. We are WELS Lutherans and have lots of peace and hope in a crazy world because of our Savior, Jesus. If you'd like to know more about our faith, visit www.wels.net. Their "Topical Q & A" page might be helpful if you have specific questions.

I am a part-time physical therapist, stay-at-home-mom, and owner, author, and publisher at Goose Water Press LLC.

Subscribe to my monthly newsletter

In order to keep in touch, I hope you'll consider joining my mailing list, which you can find at www.kristenemilybehl.com. I won't flood your inbox—I promise! It's a great way to keep you updated on what I'm working on roughly once a month, and for you to share your thoughts with me, too. Sometimes I'll ask your advice. Sometimes I'll give you a glimpse into my writing or a sneak peek at a coming manuscript or cover design. I'll share project updates, personal updates, and books I have enjoyed reading. My mailing list is the best way to make sure we can stay connected.

Leave a review

One of the most helpful things you can do for me is to leave a review! Reviews are so vital for potential readers to know whether or not they should trust me to provide them value. It would mean so much to me if you would take a moment to tell them what you think. I'd really appreciate it!

Acknowledgements

PUBLISHING A BOOK WAS A PIPE DREAM from my childhood—something I yearned to accomplish, but never thought was actually possible. It's surreal for me to hold this book in my hand. A beautiful, professional, intimately personal product. It has been far from a solitary effort. I have a lot of people to thank for helping to make this dream a reality.

First, to my husband, Phil. You were the first person to whom I revealed my passion for writing as an adult, with a real vision of actually getting something published. To you, this came out of nowhere! Thank you for not only *not* laughing at me (at least on the outside), but for supporting my passion more than I ever imagined. This meant giving up a lot of time, energy, and even some finances for the sake of my writing. Thank you for helping me to be confident in my work and own the idea of being an author. Thank you for your willingness to always listen and offer honest advice as I continue to navigate this new business of creativity. I am grateful to you beyond words. I love you more than mountains!

To the two precious little girls who made me a mama—my *real* dream come true. Thank you for teaching me so many things, and for being the source of inspiration for most of my writing these days. You have rekindled my creativity and opened new worlds I never saw coming. I love you girls more than I ever thought possible.

To a few close friends—Anne, Lauren, Bri, and Allie—who cheered me on and gave invaluable feedback on my manuscript and business plan as a whole. Thank you all for being teammates on my bench, subbing in at so many points in my life; for giving me encouragement and amazing friendship throughout high school, college, young adulthood, and motherhood. I hope I have and continue to do the same for each of you. Your friendship is a true gift.

To Anne—the same Anne!—for the amazing doodle work throughout this book and the creative suggestion to include them in the first place. I can honestly say this book wouldn't be quite what it is without you. I am so grateful for the time and effort you spent (in the limited spaces between taking care of your own job and family) to help me make this dream successful. I'm also grateful to you for giving me that original "Unsolicited Advice for the New Mama" note that meant so much to me during my first postpartum experience. To say you are a truly great friend doesn't seem to cover it.

To my family, both the Behl's and the Reiff's. You have no idea how much it meant to me when you cheered at the first mention of my writing and publishing goals. Your support rocketed me into full I-can-really-do-this mode! God has surrounded me with some truly beautiful souls. You all mean so much to me—more than I can say.

To my one and only sister, Nicole, for your constant support. You never seem phased by my new ideas. Instead, your steady calmness never hesitates to back me up, to encourage me, and to make me feel like I am capable of anything. Your belief in me is unwavering, and you have no idea how much it means to me. You're the best, sister, and I love you!

To Dan Madson, my copyeditor. You taught me so much about the difference between writing how I speak and writing to be read. I'm so thankful to you for helping me become a better writer. It's also been so uplifting to have a mentor who understands the trials and triumphs in the journey of self-publishing. I thank God for our friendship!

To David Miles, who took care of my cover design and interior formatting. Thank you for your willingness to take on a newbie and for patiently answering my many, many questions. Your designs have created a completely beautiful product that I am so proud of.

To all of the mamas who were there for me during my own pregnancy and postpartum story. Your concern and encouragement in just the right moments meant more to me than you'll ever know, and has inspired me to want to do that for others. This includes my own mom, Debbie, and my mother-in-law, Chris. Thanks for always knowing what I needed, for your relentless willingness to help, and for showing me how a strong Christian mama should be.

Most of all, I thank my God who makes all of this possible. He blesses me with both earthly and heavenly treasures that continue to astound me every day. His grace is unfailing. I hope that my work leads others to Him, to experience the peace and joy that I have as His child. Every day on this earth with the ones we love is a precious gift, but none so marvelous as the gift of eternal life that awaits us in heaven. It truly is the purpose for everything. To God be the glory!

And, of course, to my readers! If you are reading this, it means my dream of putting my work into the hands of someone who wants it has come true. I can't express to you how grateful I am that you have supported me in this way. I hope you were blessed by it and that it gave you something you craved. God bless you and your growing family!

Much love,

Kristen

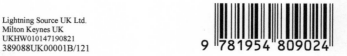